Department of Veterans Affairs
Health Services Research & Development Service | Evidence-based Synthesis Program

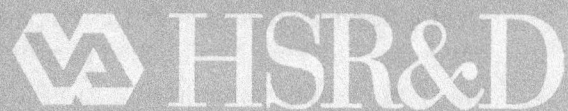

# Health Effects of Military Service on Women Veterans

May 2011

**Prepared for:**
Department of Veterans Affairs
Veterans Health Administration
Health Services Research & Development Service
Washington, DC 20420

**Prepared by:**
Evidence-based Synthesis Program (ESP) Center
West Los Angeles VA Medical Center
Los Angeles, CA
Paul G. Shekelle, M.D., Ph.D., Director

**Investigators:**
Principal Investigator:
    Paul G. Shekelle, M.D., Ph.D.

Co-Investigators:
    Fatma Batuman, M.D.
    Bevanne Bean-Mayberry, M.D., M.H.S.
    Caroline Goldzweig, M.D., M.S.P.H.
    Christine Huang, M.D.
    Donna L. Washington, M.D., M.P.H.
    Elizabeth M. Yano, PhD, M.S.P.H.
    Laurie C. Zephyrin, M.D., M.P.H., M.B.A.

Research Associate:
    Isomi M. Miake-Lye, B.A.

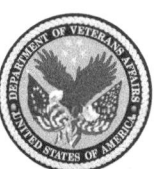

# PREFACE

Health Services Research & Development Service's (HSR&D's) Evidence-based Synthesis Program (ESP) was established to provide timely and accurate syntheses of targeted healthcare topics of particular importance to VA managers and policymakers, as they work to improve the health and healthcare of Veterans. The ESP disseminates these reports throughout VA.

HSR&D provides funding for four ESP Centers and each Center has an active VA affiliation. The ESP Centers generate evidence syntheses on important clinical practice topics, and these reports help:

- develop clinical policies informed by evidence,

- guide the implementation of effective services to improve patient outcomes and to support VA clinical practice guidelines and performance measures, and

- set the direction for future research to address gaps in clinical knowledge.

In 2009, an ESP Coordinating Center was created to expand the capacity of HSR&D Central Office and the four ESP sites by developing and maintaining program processes. In addition, the Center established a Steering Committee comprised of HSR&D field-based investigators, VA Patient Care Services, Office of Quality and Performance, and Veterans Integrated Service Networks (VISN) Clinical Management Officers. The Steering Committee provides program oversight and guides strategic planning, coordinates dissemination activities, and develops collaborations with VA leadership to identify new ESP topics of importance to Veterans and the VA healthcare system.

Comments on this evidence report are welcome and can be sent to Nicole Floyd, ESP Coordinating Center Program Manager, at nicole.floyd@va.gov.

**Recommended citation:,** Batuman F, Bean-Mayberry B, Goldzweig CL, Huang C, Miake-Lye IM, Washington DL, Yano EM, Zephyrin LC, Shekelle PG. Health Effects of Military Service on Women Veterans. VA-ESP Project # 05-226; 2011.

This report is based on research conducted by the Evidence-based Synthesis Program (ESP) Center located at the West Los Angeles VA Medical Center, Los Angeles, CA funded by the Department of Veterans Affairs, Veterans Health Administration, Office of Research and Development, Health Services Research and Development. The findings and conclusions in this document are those of the author(s) who are responsible for its contents; the findings and conclusions do not necessarily represent the views of the Department of Veterans Affairs or the United States government. Therefore, no statement in this article should be construed as an official position of the Department of Veterans Affairs. No investigators have any affiliations or financial involvement (e.g., employment, consultancies, honoraria, stock ownership or options, expert testimony, grants or patents received or pending, or royalties) that conflict with material presented in the report.

# TABLE OF CONTENTS

# EXECUTIVE SUMMARY

## BACKGROUND

In response to a growing need to understand the effects of military service on health status, this report supplements our prior review by focusing directly on the reproductive and trauma effects on women in the military or Veterans who have been deployed. The goal is to broaden the knowledge of VA policy leaders and clinicians about post-deployment health issues for women.

The Key Questions were:

Key Question #1: What research has been published on the effects of deployment on post-deployment reproductive outcomes?

We operationalized "reproductive effects" to encompass the following: fertility issues, birth defects, menstrual effects (e.g., change in cycles, loss of cycles), urinary tract infections, sexually transmitted infections, and reproductive cancers (e.g., cervical, ovarian, etc).

Key Question #2: What research has been published on post-trauma sequelae in OEF/OIF women Veterans, including: mental health problems, suicide, cardiovascular disease, risky health behaviors (including: tobacco use, hazardous alcohol use, substance abuse, suicide, homicide, assaultive behavior, and eating disorders), and other post-trauma sequelae?

## METHODS

We searched PubMed in August 2010 using standard search terms. Titles, abstracts, and articles were reviewed in duplicate by team members trained in the critical analysis of literature. Articles were classified according to subject category and narratively summarized in evidence tables.

## RESULTS

We screened 2,359 titles, rejected 2,302 based on systematic criteria, and performed a more detailed review of 57 articles that met criteria. From these, we identified 15 articles relating to Key Question #1 (post-deployment reproductive effects) and 29 relating to Key Question #2 (post-trauma sequelae among OEF/OIF women Veterans).

### Key Question #1. What research has been published on the effects of deployment on post-deployment reproductive outcomes?

The evidence base for reproductive effects of deployment of women Veterans is modest, mostly consisting of single studies of specific deployments and particular outcomes. Of note, there have been no published assessments of reproductive effects of the current (since 2003) deployments. Data about reproductive effects from past deployments are insufficient to reach strong conclusions. Because many of the outcomes of interest (birth defects, gynecologic cancers) are rare, large sample sizes are needed to assess for possible associations, and often times response rates for large sample studies are below desirable levels. This makes the interpretation of findings questionable.

**Key Question #2. What research has been published on post-trauma sequelae in OEF/OIF women Veterans, including: mental health problems, suicide, cardiovascular disease, risky health behaviors (including: tobacco use, hazardous alcohol use, substance abuse, suicide, homicide, assaultive behavior, and eating disorders), and other post-trauma sequelae?**

The 13 publications focusing on the post-deployment mental health of our OEF/OIF Veterans found increased risks for new-onset depression, suicide, and firearm suicide; discrepancy between the mental health needs and utilization of mental health services, greater risks for mental disorder hospitalizations, and higher utilization of non-mental health medical services among Veterans with mental health diagnoses; and higher risks for mental diagnoses among certain subgroups.

The post-trauma sequelae highlights three visible issues: 1) early TBI data show a preponderance of men from the military; ongoing evaluation is needed to understand what, if any, gender issues may be important for ongoing care; 2) alcohol use in recently returning women Veterans presents greater risk at lower levels of consumption for women with other risk conditions (PTSD MST, combat trauma); and 3) health care utilization by gender and diagnosis requires ongoing follow-up because while women may initiate contact with VA sooner, utilization did not differ. Moreover, conditions examined so far for deployed or post-deployed women manifest differently (pain syndromes) or differ in cause for evacuation from theatre. Individual studies also examined a number of other possible associations, such as eating disorders, pain, post-deployment distress, etc.; data are too sparse to draw firm conclusions.

## CONCLUSIONS

With the continued expansion of women's role in the military, better understanding of the potential health effects of military service on women during and after their miltary service is essential. While the emerging literature in this area is relatively limited to date, several important themes are nonetheless apparent.

The evidence on the influence of military service on reproductive health is mixed and relies on a modest literature base. Generally, pregnancy outcomes do not appear to differ among deployed vs. undeployed women. However, while several studies demonstrate non-significant differences by deployment status, others present contradictory evidence on the influence of military service on rates of spontaneous abortion, stillbirths, and ectopic pregnancies. Influences on birth outcomes raise more questions than they answer. Only one study reported birthweights, which did not appear to differ by deployment experience of their mothers. More studies have focused on birth defects: about half indicate there are no significant differences in birth defect rates among deployed vs. non-deployed women, whereas the other half report higher rates that are not statistically significant (reflecting problems in statistical power associated with sample sizes for these rare events) or in fact reflect higher rates.

The evidence on post-trauma sequellae among OEF/OIF women (soldiers and Veterans) is also relatively limited, and reflects a chief emphasis on mental health issues. Most of these studies are descriptive, and allude to gender differences in diagnosis, impact and health care utilization. Depression and suicide are major foci, demonstrating the highest rates of incident depression among women who are deployed and also exposed to combat. Interestingly, deployment without such exposure was associated with lower rates of incident depression than non-deployment. Women Veterans also had higher risks for depression than men, though lower substance use disorders. Suicide risk was reported as being lower among women Veterans, but the standardized mortality ratio among female Veterans is reportedly higher than that of male Veterans. Several of these studies focused on the differences among Veterans vs. non-Veterans more than women vs. men. For example, the suicide rate among all Veterans (male and female) is estimated to be 66 percent higher than that of the general population. Also, among suicide decedents, women Veterans were 1.6 times more likely to use firearms (compared to non-Veterans).

The literature on mental health needs and utilization among OEF/OIF women Veterans was also descriptive and limited. Younger women Veterans were less likely than young male Veterans to use mental health services, which was in contrast to older Veterans (i.e., older women Veterans were more likely to use mental health services than older male Veterans). This pattern held overall and for those with substance abuse or mood/anxiety disorders, whereas no gender differences were found for PTSD care-seeking. Female soldiers had higher risks of hospitalization for mental disorders, and were more likely to be psychiatric evacuees from the field.

The remainder of the literature on other post-trauma sequelae was variable in topic. The evidence of problem-drinking among OEF/OIF women Veterans is mixed (two studies which present contradictory findings). Some of this literature focuses on examing gender differences. For example, predictors of women Veterans' readmission rates for inpatient drug treatment include sexual and physical abuse before, during and after deployment (vs. substance abuse, aggression, and cognitive impairment among men). OEF/OIF women had higher rates of military sexual trauma (MST); and women with MST used VA care more, were less satisfied and had lower perceptions of VA facilities and staff, with particular problems with VA staff among those who had also had combat exposure. OEF/OIF women were less likely to witness the level of killing that men experienced and were less likely to have traumatic brain injuries (TBI), compared to men. Effects of deployment among OEF/OIF women included higher rates of moderate to severe pain, higher distress after the first deployment, and, when added with combat experiences, high rates of eating disorders and extreme weight loss.

## FUTURE RESEARCH

In summary, differential effects of military service by gender are apparent, though the volume and quality of the literature is as yet modest. Given that the published scientific literature not uncommonly reflects prior years' research investment in different topic areas, we anticipate that the investment in women's health research by the U.S. Departments of Veterans Affairs and Defense will contribute to a rapidly growing literature base on the health effects of military service on women over the next several years. Such growth may warrant an updated systematic review, comparable to the overarching review that was recently updated,[4] which demonstrated that more articles were published between 2004 and 2008 than the previous 25 years combined.

More research is needed on the reproductive health effects of military service. Currently, the evidence is mixed with respect to impacts on pregnancy and birth outcomes. One case control study reported an association between rates of birth defects and deployment status, begging the question about what elements of military service (or pursuit of service) might be contributing factors. The available literature also lacks descriptive evidence of the range of reproductive health issues that women in the military and women Veterans face. Currently, there are studies in progress that may well contribute substantively to this knowledge base, but that are not yet in the published literature.

The VA research portfolio on OEF/OIF Veterans' health and health care will also contribute to the emerging literature on the consequences of military service among OEF/OIF women Veterans. The current literature lays some of the groundwork but does so less comprehensively (spanning topics of mental health, physical health, social function, and so on) than would be optimal. Future research should begin to fill these gaps to produce an increasingly detailed portrait of their post-trauma sequelae.

# EVIDENCE REPORT

## INTRODUCTION

### BACKGROUND

Women Veterans are among the fastest growing groups of new VA health care users of the VA healthcare system, and currently reflect approximately eight percent of all U.S. Veterans. With Operation Enduring Freedom and Iraqi Freedom (OEF/OIF), women comprise a larger percentage of the military (11.3 percent) than of prior military operations. As of fiscal year 2010, 51.3 percent of female OEF/OIF Veterans had enrolled in VA health care, in sharp contrast to women from previous eras (an estimated 11 percent). Of this group, 88 percent have used VA health care more than once.[1]

To better understand the needs of this rapidly growing group, women Veterans' health research has expanded as well.[2] Two previous systematic reviews examined the literature on women Veterans' health and health care up to 2008.[3, 4] In this review, we specifically explored women Veterans' post-deployment health, with two main areas of concentration: 1) post-deployment effects on reproductive health for women Veterans, and 2) post-trauma sequelae among women Veterans from the OEF/OIF cohort.

The published literature on deployment and post-deployment health was included in the two previous systematic literature reviews. Most of the extant literature focused on the population of Veterans from OEF/OIF. The previous review also examined the reproductive health literature among military women and women Veterans. However, the previous reviews assessed the literature up through 2008, while the current review further updates these topics by examining them in more detail and extending the literature search through 2010.

# METHODS

## TOPIC DEVELOPMENT

This project was nominated by Patricia Hayes, PhD, Chief Consultant for the Women Veterans Health Strategic Health Care Group, with input from a technical expert panel.

The final key questions are:

Key Question #1: What research has been published on the effects of deployment on post-deployment reproductive outcomes?

We operationalized "reproductive effects" to encompass the following: fertility issues, birth defects, menstrual effects (e.g., change in cycles, loss of cycles), urinary tract infections, sexually transmitted infections, and reproductive cancers (e.g., cervical, ovarian, etc).

Key Question #2: What research has been published on post-trauma sequelae in OEF/OIF women Veterans, including: mental health problems, suicide, cardiovascular disease, risky health behaviors (including: tobacco use, hazardous alcohol use, substance abuse, homicide, assaultive behavior, and eating disorders), and other post-trauma sequelae?

## SEARCH STRATEGY

The broader topic of research on women Veterans' health has been the subject of two previous systematic reviews from our group. Those reviews included articles meeting our eligibility criteria through the end of their respective search dates. Goldzweig et al. (2006)[3] covered women Veterans' health and health care issues through 2004. In that systematic review, we identified 182 studies, including two randomized controlled studies and 180 studies with observational designs. Bean-Mayberry et al. (2010)[4] updated the Goldzweig et al. search from 2004 through 2008. In that review, we identified 195 articles, with five articles describing results of randomized controlled trials. We assessed the original articles identified in these reviews for eligibility for inclusion in the current systematic review (as described below). We also developed a search strategy specific to the key questions for this review, covering the period from 2008 to the present. The search terms and Medical Subject Headings (MeSH) for the various search strategies are found in Appendix 1. Searches were conducted through August 2010.

## STUDY SELECTION

Two team members (IML and PGS) reviewed the list of titles and selected articles for further review. Eligible articles had as their subject U.S. women Veterans, with a clear indication that they had been deployed, and reported outcomes on reproductive effects (including fertility issues, birth defects, menstrual effects, urinary tract infections, sexually transmitted diseases, and reproductive cancers); or had as their subject U.S. women Veterans of OEF/OIF and reported outcomes on post-trauma sequelae. Post-trauma sequelae included mental health problems, suicide, cardiovascular disease, risky health behaviors (including tobacco use, hazardous alcohol use, substance abuse, homicide, assaultive behavior, and eating disorders), and other post-trauma sequelae.

Because reviews of the effects of Agent Orange[5] and Gulf War Syndrome[6] already exist, we did not review their effects in any more detail in this review. Similarly, in our prior reports, we devoted sections to the literature on military sexual trauma (MST) and post-traumatic stress disorder (PTSD), and did not repeat that information here.

Because of the emerging nature of this particular literature, we did not require any restrictions on study design. Therefore, this review includes a wide range of observational and descriptive studies.

## DATA ABSTRACTION

We abstracted the following data from included studies: sample characteristics, sample size, design, objectives, main measures, and main findings.

## DATA SYNTHESIS

We constructed evidence tables showing the study characteristics and results for all included studies, organized by key question. (See Appendix 2 and Appendix 3.) We analyzed studies to compare their characteristics, methods, and findings. We compiled a summary of findings for each key question or clinical topic, and drew conclusions based on qualitative synthesis of the findings.

## PEER REVIEW

A draft version of this report was sent to five peer reviewers and the report was extensively revised based on their input.

# RESULTS

## LITERATURE FLOW

The combined library contained 2,452 citations, of which we reviewed 57 articles at the full-text level. From these, we identified eligible studies that addressed one of the key questions. For Key Question #1, we found 15 studies; and for Key Question #2, we found 29. We grouped the studies by key question, and within each key question by topic area.

## KEY QUESTION #1. What research has been published on post-deployment reproductive effects in any deployment of women Veterans?

We identified 15 articles[7-21] that assessed the post-deployment effects on reproductive health for women Veterans. Two were about Vietnam Veterans[9, 10] and 13 were about Gulf War Veterans.[7,8,11-21] There were two cases where there was more than one study assessing a particular post-deployment effect for a particular war: there were two studies that assessed gender-specific effects in Gulf War Veterans,[7, 19] and eight studies that assessed the frequency of birth defects following the Gulf War.[9,11-14,16,18,20]

### Gynecologic Cancer – Vietnam Women Veterans

Kang et al. studied the prevalence of gynecologic cancers among female Vietnam Veterans.[10] In this study, 4,140 female Vietnam Veterans and 4,140 female Veteran controls from other military eras completed a structured telephone interview regarding any history of gynecologic cancer. As a measure of association between the risk of cancer and military service in Vietnam, odds ratios and 95 percent confidence intervals were calculated using multiple logistic regression models that yielded estimates of potential confounders. Data revealed that 8 percent of Vietnam Veterans and 7.1 percent of non-Vietnam Veterans reported a history of gynecologic cancers (breast, ovary, uterus, and cervix), but this difference was not statistically significant. Female Vietnam Veterans have not experienced a higher prevalence of gynecologic cancer in the 30 years since the conflict.

### Sexual Function – Gulf War Women Veterans

In a case control study, Gilhooly et al. compared female sexual dysfunction in female Gulf War Veterans with or without chronic fatigue syndrome.[15] The 26 female Veterans with symptoms consonant with chronic fatigue syndrome, as assessed in an enrollment questionnaire, were compared to 22 female Veterans without indications of chronic fatigue syndrome. Those with chronic fatigue had worse sexual dysfunction (defined as a positive response to a query about generalized difficulty with sexual function) than the 22 female Veterans without chronic fatigue syndrome (60 percent vs. 10 percent, p,.002). Of note, many of the subjects with chronic fatigue also had Axis I psychiatric disorders.

**Figure 1. Literature Flow Chart**

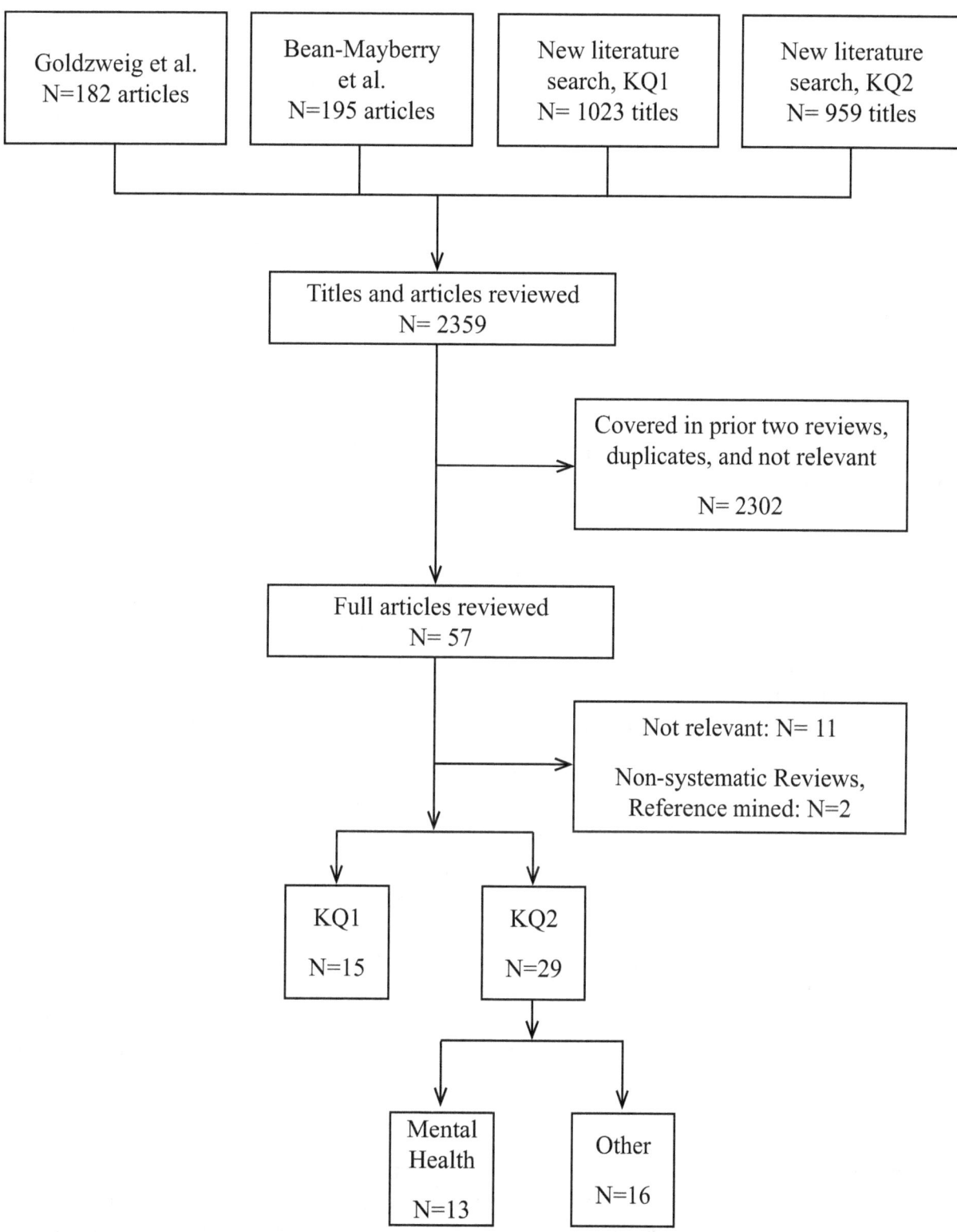

## Conception/Fertility/Pregnancy

### Vietnam Women Veterans

Kang et al.[9] analyzed pregnancy outcomes among female Vietnam Veterans in a case control study. The cohort study compared self reported pregnancy outcomes for 4,140 female Vietnam Veterans with those of 4,140 non-deployed female Veterans. As a measure of association, they calculated odd ratios and 95 percent confidence intervals using logistic regression adjusting for age at conception, race, education, military nursing status, smoking, drinking, and other exposures during pregnancy. There was no statistically significant association between military service in Vietnam and adverse pregnancy outcomes (i.e., spontaneous abortion, low birth weight, or pre-term delivery). However, the risk of likely or moderate to severe birth defects (i.e., likely defects included congenital anomalies and included structural, functional, metabolic or hereditary defects) was significantly higher among Vietnam Veterans versus non-Vietnam Veterans (10.5 percent vs. 7.0 percent and 7.7 percent vs 5.8 percent respectively).

### Gulf War Women Veterans

Araneta et al. studied conception and pregnancy during the Persian Gulf War and the risk to female Veterans. 1,558 completed (response rate 50 percent, of an original sample of 3,105) the questionnaire.[7] Self-reported reproductive outcomes and dates, gestational data, and individual deployment dates identified 415 Gulf War exposed pregnancies, 298 Gulf War Veteran postwar conceptions, and 427 non-deployed women Veteran pregnancies. Pregnancy outcomes for Gulf War exposed conceptions and non-deployed conceptions were similar. However, spontaneous abortions and ectopic pregnancies were elevated for Gulf War Veterans who conceived postwar. Specifically, in the adjusted analyses, GWV postwar conceptions had a three-fold risk of spontaneous abortion (adjusted OR 2.92, 95% CI 1.9, 4.6) and nearly an eight times higher risk of ectopic pregnancy (adjusted OR 7.70, 95% CI 3.0, 19.8) compared to non-deployed Veterans.

A similar study was performed by Wells and colleagues.[19] These authors sampled 20,000 subjects from the Defense Manpower Data Center, equally divided between men and women, who were either deployed or non-deployed Veterans during the 1991 Gulf War, who were married, and who were between the ages 18 and 33. The response rate to a survey about reproductive issues was 51 percent (8,742 out of 17,140 with valid addresses). Among 2,235 female and 2,159 male participants there were no differences in birth weight outcomes between Gulf War and non-deployed Veterans. As opposed to the results of Araneta and colleagues,[7] this study found no differences between groups in the risk for ectopic pregnancies, stillbirths, or miscarriages. The reasons for the discrepancy in results between the two studies are unclear. Both studies had lower-than-desired response rates (about 50 percent for each), and perhaps the discrepant results merely reflect the experience of the Veterans who elected to respond to the surveys.

## Birth Defects

Penman 1996[18] used population based registries to examine birth defects and live-born and stillborn children born to men and women in two National Guard units in southeast Mississippi who were deployed from August 1990 through July 1991. From these two units, 54 children were compared to the birth defect rates observed in the general public, using the following birth defect surveillance systems: Metropolitan Atlanta Congenital Defects Program, the Centers for Disease Control's Birth Defects Monitoring Program, and the California Birth Defects Monitoring

Program. They concluded that the observed number of birth defects among children conceived by and born to this group of Persian Gulf War Veterans was not greater than expected on the basis of population-based registries.

Cowan 1997[14] compared the overall risk of birth defects among 33,998 infants born to GWV and 41,463 infants born to non deployed Veterans (NDV) at 135 military hospitals between 1991 and 1993. In this study, there was no increase in birth defects among children of GWV. The prevalence of any birth defect was 7.45 percent for deployed Veterans and 7.59 percent for non-deployed Veterans (RR 0.98, 95% CI 0.93-1.03). There was no significant association between service in the Gulf War and the prevalence of any birth defect for male Veterans (OR 0.97, 95% CI 0.91-1.03) or female Veterans (OR 1.07, 95% CI 0.94-1.22) even after adjustment for mother's age at delivery, race or ethnicity, and marital status of parent at the time of the Gulf War. This article is significant for its large sample size, use of medical record data to ascertain the outcomes of interest, and its multivariable analysis that included adjusting for multiple potential confounders.

Araneta 2000[12] studied offspring born to Gulf War Veterans (GWV) and non-deployed Veterans (NDV) by cross-referencing personal records of military personnel with birth certificates and the Hawaii Birth Defects Program records between 1989 and 1993. The pilot study identified 17,182 military infants of GWV and 13,465 infants of NDV in Hawaii and compared prevalence congenital anomalies through the first year of life. In this study, the prevalence of 48 birth defects was similar in NDV and GWV groups in conceptions that happened before the war and conceptions during and after the Gulf War. This study was limited by small numbers of case infants with birth defects and thus did not have adequate statistical power for rare defects. Additionally, they were unable to evaluate the role of maternal GWV exposure because of the small numbers of births in female GWV (165 births) in Hawaii.

Araneta 2003[13] expanded the study to include infants born to Gulf War Veterans (GWV) and non-deployed Veterans registered in Arkansas, Arizona, California, Georgia, Hawaii and Iowa Birth Defects Program in 1989 to 1993. The sample size was 11,961 infants of GWV and 33,052 infants of NVD. Approximately 4,400 infants were born to women Veterans, and of these 450 infants were born to women Veterans who had been deployed in the Gulf War. Among 308 infants born to GWV women after the war, compared to 1,959 infants born to non-deployed women Veterans, the only difference that was statistically significant was the frequency of hypospadius and epispadius (4 cases among 308 in GWV and 4 cases among 1,959 non-deployed Veterans, Relative Risk = 6.4, 95% CI = 1.5, 26.8). However, for 47 other defects, no statistically significant differences were found. These data were unadjusted for potential confounders. Parenthetically, the study found in male GWV a higher incidence in various cardiac valve defects in offspring.

Werler 2004[20] identified cases from craniofacial centers in 26 cities (US and Canada). In specific, this study was concerned with a potential effect of military service on the risk of offspring with hemifacial microsomia, also known as Goldenhar syndrome. There were 232 cases of infants with Goldenhar syndrome and 832 controls ascertained from the pediatricians of cases or from a similar practice, and matched within two months of the birth date of the case. The birth year of cases and controls were between 1996 and 2002. There were no statistically significantly increased odds of Goldenhar syndrome in multivariable analyses for military service by either mother or father, or by any parent having served in the Gulf War. There was a statistically significant association for any parent being in the Army (adjusted odds ratio = 2.4, 95% CI 1.4, 4.21); however, this study does not provide evidence supporting an association between Gulf War service and the presence of Goldenhar syndrome.

Langlois 2009[11] reported on a population based case control study assessing 30 major birth defects. The study is national and contains data on military service. In analyses adjusted for maternal age, race/ethnicity and education, there was no statistically significant association for any of the 30 major birth defects and military service since 1990, for infants born between 1997 and 2003. However, due to the small numbers of parents reporting military service, the 95 percent confidence interval in most estimates are wide (for example, among 202 cases of spina bifida, there were three mothers with military service for a rate of 1.5 percent, compared with a rate of 1.1 percent of control infants whose mothers had military service, yielding an adjusted odds ratio of 0.72, 95% CI 0.26, 2.01).

A study by Kane et al,[9] previously discussed in the conception/fertility/pregnancy section, also assessed the association of Vietnam deployment in birth defects. The authors reported that the risk of likely or moderate to severe birth defects (i.e., likely defects included congenital anomalies and included structural, functional, metabolic, or hereditary defects) was significantly higher among Vietnam Veterans versus non-Vietnam Veterans (10.5 percent vs. 7.0 percent and 7.7 percent vs. 5.8 percent, respectively).

One additional study, reported in only a few paragraphs, surveyed 11,441 Gulf War Veterans and 9,476 non-Gulf War Veterans, and there were 6,043 pregnancies.[16] The survey response rate was stated as 70 percent. Female Gulf War Veterans "reported more miscarriages and stillbirths" than non-Gulf War Veterans, but "neither [difference] was significant." No other details were presented. The author also reported that "female Gulf War Veterans were nearly three-fold likelier than control subjects to have a child with likely birth defect (adjusted O.R. 2.97, 95% CI 1.47-5.99)." Again, no additional details are reported.

## General Gynecologic/Reproductive Health

Pierce studied physical and emotional health of female Gulf War Veterans.[8] Five hundred twenty-five women participated in the study following the war and again in a follow-up study two years later (sampled from members of the Air Force: active, guard, or reserve). Measures included general physical health, gender specific health, "Gulf War Syndrome," and PTSD. Multiple statistical analyses were used to describe women's physical and emotional health at these two time points. Deployed female Veterans reported significantly more general and gender specific health problems than did women who were not deployed during that conflict. The reproductive findings included abnormal pap smears (10.4 percent vs. 4.9 percent) and breast cysts/lumps (13.4 percent vs. 6.0 percent) in women deployed to the Gulf versus other regions. Additional research is warranted to define the health effects and their etiology.

Murphy et al. studied the healthcare implications for female Veterans and active duty troops.[17] They performed a literature review using MEDLINE and collected data from VA and DOD registries. There were 49,950 female troops deployed to the Persian Gulf during Operations Desert Shield and Storm. The mean age of deployed women was the same as for men, 26.5. The most common complaints involved minor orthopedic, acute respiratory, dermatologic, dental, and acute GI problems. A similar percentage of women and men presented with these outpatient complaints. However, women made proportionally more visits to sick call than men, and 26 percent of visits by women were for gynecologic problems (uterine bleeding, amenorrhea, fungal vaginitis, and request for oral contraceptive refills were common reasons for visits by female troops). Only three percent of all visits by women required referrals to gynecologists.

Wittich[21] examined the creation of the Gulf War comprehensive clinical evaluation program at Tripler Army Medical Center. Of the first 100 Veterans seen, 16 percent were women. Half of the 16 Gulf War female Veterans experienced gynecologic problems while deployed and 43 percent have had problems since returning. There is no comparison done with non-deployed Veterans or the general population in this study. After returning from active duty, six patients became pregnant, five had normal outcomes and one had a miscarriage.

## Summary of KQ1

The evidence base for reproductive effects of deployment of women Veterans is modest, mostly consisting of single studies of specific deployments and particular outcomes. Of note, there have been no published assessments of reproductive effects of the current (since 2003) deployments. Data about reproductive effects from past deployments are insufficient to reach strong conclusions. Because many of the outcomes of interest (birth defects, gynecologic cancers) are rare, large sample sizes are needed to assess for possible associations, and often times response rates for large sample studies are below desirable levels. This makes the interpretation of findings questionable.

## KEY QUESTION #2. What research has been published on post-trauma sequelae in OEF/OIF women Veterans, including: mental health problems, suicide, cardiovascular disease, risky health behaviors (including: tobacco use, hazardous alcohol use, substance abuse, homicide, assaultive behavior, and eating disorders), and other post-trauma sequelae?

For Key Question #2, we note here that, as opposed to Key Question #1, all studies in this section concern OEF/OIF Veterans.

## Mental Health

Thirteen publications focused on mental health sequelae and covered three general areas: depression and suicide,[22-25] needs and utilization,[26-30] and risk factors for mental health diagnosis.[31-34]

### Depression and Suicide

A study by Wells and colleagues[25] prospectively investigated new-onset depression by deployment status and gender. Deployed men and women with combat exposures had the highest rates of onset of depression. Compared to non-deployed men and women, combat-deployed men and women were at increased risk for depression (men: adjusted odds ratio [AOR]=1.32; 95% CI=1.13, 1.54; women: AOR=2.13; 95% CI=1.70, 2.65), whereas deployment without combat exposures led to decreased risk (men: AOR=0.66; 95% CI=0.53, 0.83; women: AOR=0.65; 95% CI=0.47, 0.89). This study was part of the Millennium Cohort Study, and uses standardized survey questions for both outcomes and predictors.

Three studies examined suicide rates. Zivin and colleagues[22] reported on clinical and demographic factors associated with suicide among depressed Veterans. This study used data collected as part of VA's National Registry for Depression, and provides longitudinal service use data and pharmacy data for over 1.5 million Veterans diagnosed with depression since 1997. The primary outcome was suicide as defined by the National Death Index. Among 807,964 Veterans included in this study (which excluded bipolar depression, schizophrenia, schizoaffective, cases prior to 1999, among other criteria), 1,683 (0.21 percent) committed suicide. Importantly, this study, while reporting that men are at greater risk for suicide than women, found that the male-to-female ratio in VA is somewhat less (3:1) than in the general population (4:1). McCarthy and colleagues[24] compared suicide rates among Veterans to that of the general population. Overall, for men and women combined, suicide risks among Veterans Health patients were 66 percent higher than those observed in the general US population. For male patients, the crude VHA suicide rate was 43.13/100,000 person-years, compared with 23.2/100,000 person-years among males in the general population, with age-adjusted standardized mortality ratio of 1.66 (95% CI=1.58, 1.74). For female patients, the crude suicide rate was 10.41/100,000 person-years, compared with 5.22/100,000 person-years among females in the general population, with a standardized mortality ratio of 1.87 (95% CI=1.35, 2.47). Another study by Kaplan and colleagues[23] specifically examined firearm use among Veteran suicide decedents. Across the age groups, male and female Veterans had higher firearm suicide rates than non-Veterans. Among males and females, younger Veterans (18 to 34 years) had the highest firearm and total suicide rates. The male and female Veteran suicide decedents were, respectively, 1.3 and 1.6 times more likely to use firearms relative to non-Veterans after adjusting for age, marital status, race, and region of residence.

## Mental Health Care Needs and Utilization

Five studies focused on mental health care needs and utilization. Owens and colleagues[26] found that the most frequently reported concerns for which participants in this study of 50 OEF/OIF Veterans who completed an Internet survey indicated they needed counseling were depression (48 percent), relationship issues (38 percent), anxiety (36 percent), and anger management (30 percent). Although 78 percent of respondents reported that they felt they needed treatment in the past year, 42 percent of these individuals indicated that they did not seek counseling or treatment. Long waiting periods for appointments (33 percent) and prior bad experiences (28 percent) were the top two reported barriers to seeking mental health services in the VA.

In a logistic regression analysis, Chatterjee and colleagues[27] compared gender differences amongst a sample of 782,789 Veterans with at least one outpatient visit in the VA in FY99 associated with a mental health or substance abuse diagnosis and discovered that, overall, younger women Veterans (<35 years old) were significantly less likely and older women (35 to 54 years old) more likely to use any mental health services in comparison with their male counterparts. This trend held true for the subgroup of Veterans with a substance abuse (SA) or mood/anxiety disorder. However, among the subgroup of Veterans with PTSD or a bipolar/psychotic disorder, there were no significant gender differences in the likelihood of utilizing mental health services. Among men and women Veterans 55 or older, there were no significant differences in utilization within diagnostic categories.

In a study by Seal and colleagues,[35] of 49,425 Veterans with newly diagnosed PTSD, only 9.5 percent attended nine or more VA mental health sessions in 15 weeks or less in the first year of diagnosis. Engagement in nine or more VA treatment sessions for PTSD within 15 weeks varied by predisposing variables (age and gender), enabling variables (clinic of first mental health diagnosis and distance from VA facility), and need (type and complexity of mental health diagnoses). Only a minority of Iraq and Afghanistan Veterans with new PTSD diagnoses received the recommended number and intensity of VA mental health treatment sessions within the first year of diagnosis.

A retrospective study by Wojcik and colleagues[30] of 473,964 U.S. Army soldiers deployed to Iraq and Afghanistan through December 2004 examined mental disorder hospitalizations, with a total of 1,948 psychiatric hospitalizations of deployed soldiers. The most common mental problems were mood, adjustment, anxiety, and substance-abuse related disorders. Both female soldiers and enlisted soldiers had significantly greater risks for mental disorder hospitalizations in both OIF and OEF operations as compared to their male and non-enlisted counterparts, with relative risks of ranging from 1.6 to 3, and 2 to 6, respectively. Younger women had the highest incidence of attempted suicide/self-inflicted injuries.

 The fifth study by Cohen and colleagues[28] compared utilization of VA non-mental health medical services across three groups of Iraq and Afghanistan Veterans: those without mental disorders, those with mental disorders other than PTSD, and those with PTSD. Veterans with mental health diagnoses, particularly PTSD, had significantly greater utilization of non-mental health medical services. Female sex and lower rank were also independently associated with greater utilization.

*Risk Factors for Mental Health Diagnosis*

Four studies focused on risk factors for mental health diagnoses or the development of mental health disorders. Rundell and colleagues[31] characterized 1,264 OEF and OIF military personnel who were psychiatrically evacuated from the theater of operations. When compared with all returned OEF/OIF Veterans, psychiatric evacuees were more likely to be: female, under the age of 31 years, African-American or Hispanic, enlisted or National Guard/Reserve. Over 80 percent of patients were evacuated during the first six months, compared with 17 percent during the second six months of deployment.

In a study of 289,328 Iraq and Afghanistan Veterans by Seal and colleagues,[32] 36.9 percent of the Iraq and Afghanistan Veterans received mental health diagnoses, including 21.8 percent with new PTSD diagnoses followed by 17.4 percent with depression diagnoses. Adjusted two-year prevalence rates of PTSD increased four to seven times after the invasion of Iraq. Active duty Veterans younger than 25 years had higher rates of PTSD and alcohol and drug use disorder diagnoses compared with active duty Veterans older than 40 years (adjusted relative risk = 2.0 and 4.9, respectively). Women were at higher risk for depression than were men, but men had over twice the risk for drug use disorders. Greater combat exposure was associated with higher risk for PTSD. Baker and colleagues[33] found that only a minority (36 percent) of their study OEF/OIF Veterans and reservists who enrolled at the VA San Diego Healthcare System did not screen positive for mental health symptoms; the remainder met threshold PTSD, depression, or substance and alcohol abuse. Gender, age, race, and rank were not significantly related to PTSD; whereas most recent branch of service and report of injury during combat were.

An additional literature review by Street and colleagues[34] highlights the emerging issues relevant to the development of PTSD among women deployed to Iraq and Afghanistan. The review explores gender differences in combat experiences and in PTSD following combat exposure; sexual assault, sexual harassment, and other interpersonal stressors experienced during deployment; women Veterans' premilitary trauma exposure; and unique stressors faced by women Veterans during the homecoming readjustment period. The authors conclude that gender-specific risk of PTSD differs substantially by type of traumatic event.

### Summary of Mental Health Post-Trauma Sequelae

The above 13 publications focusing on the post-deployment mental health of our OEF/OIF Veterans found increased risks for new-onset depression, suicide, and firearm suicide; discrepancy between the mental health needs and utilization of mental health services, greater risks for mental disorder hospitalizations, and higher utilization of non-mental health medical services among Veterans with mental health diagnoses; and higher risks for mental diagnoses among certain subgroups.

## Other Post-trauma Sequelae

Sixteen publications focused on post-trauma sequelae in areas other than mental health. These include: spinal cord injury and disorder and traumatic brain injury,[36-38] alcohol and substance abuse,[39-41] health assessments and tools related to post-trauma sequelae,[42-44] general health concerns,[45-48] and miscellaneous post-trauma sequelae.[49-51]

### Spinal Cord Injury and Disorder (SCI&D) and Traumatic Brain Injury (TBI)

The first study of 8,983 unique SCI&D users of VA health care during 2001 focused on geographical distance as a VA barrier to care?[36]. LaVela et al. found that patients in general used outpatient services less frequently when VA facilities were farther from their residence; however, male Veterans were less likely than female Veterans to use outpatient care (i.e., fewer annual visits). However, in this population of all SCI&D Veterans, women comprised only two percent of the sample and further studies are warranted to confirm and understand trends in utilization patterns for this subgroup. Loney[37] examined war wounded (n = 47) and non-war wounded (n = 72) men and women aged 18 years and older with TBI in a retrospective cohort study and noted that those with war injuries versus non-war injuries experienced lower functional scores and took longer periods to transition to rehabilitation centers. This study included 10 women. Additionally, Bell[38] looked at closed and penetrating TBI and found that most head injuries admitted to military hospitals were in males (98 percent), and most types consisted of penetrating brain injuries due to blast explosions.

### Alcohol and Substance Abuse

In the substance abuse literature, alcohol misuse was greater among OEF/OIF young men compared to non-OEF/OIF men and either group of women. No difference in rates of alcohol misuse was present for the two groups of OEF/OIF and non-OEF/OIF women.[40] However, in an OEF/OIF sample of women Veterans who had positive PTSD symptoms, 47 percent screened positive for high risk drinking.[41] Separately, re-admission rates for inpatient drug treatment differed among women and men Veterans.[39] Sexual and physical abuse in childhood, the military, or prior two years were the most potent predictors of readmission for women while substance abuse, aggression, and cognitive impairment were potent predictors for men.

### Health Assessments and Tools

For studies evaluating health assessments and tools, females were less likely to report health changes on Post Deployment Health Assessments,[43] and the Post Deployment Readjustment Inventory combined with other tools found that type of war exposures differed by gender.[42] Women reported a higher rate of MST than men, and men reported a higher rate of witnessing others injured or killed than women.[42] Fitzgerald[44] provided a primary care nurse practitioner guide for screening women Veterans in civilian primary care settings for post-traumatic stress disorder (PTSD), traumatic brain injury (TBI), and military sexual trauma (MST) with supportive data for each screening tool described and with the recommendation for accurate diagnosis and treatment of women Veterans who might be seen for routine care.

### General Health Concerns

For post-deployment general health concerns, four articles involving women OEF/OIF Veterans were identified.[45-48] One study indicated that first time deployments were associated with increased post-deployment distress in men and women, while the association between increased deployment length and post-deployment distress was found for men only.[45] However, women deployed with combat exposures were 1.78 times more likely to develop disordered eating and 2.35 times more likely to lose an extreme amount of weight when compared with women who deployed but did not report combat exposures.[48] For returning OEF/OIF Veterans, women were more likely to use outpatient services, but once initiated the frequency of visits over time did not differ by gender.[46] For returning OEF/OIF Veterans using VA care, women were less likely to report any pain, compared to male Veterans. For those with pain, women were more likely to report moderate to severe pain, but were less likely to report persistent pain compared to men Veterans.[47]

### Miscellaneous Post-Trauma Sequelae

Lastly, we identified three eligible studies that did not fit any of our existing categories; they are described here. The first[49] identifies more health care use, less satisfaction and poorer perceptions of VHA facilities and staff among women with a history of military sexual trauma. Of the 1,496 participants, 288 reported that they experienced military sexual assault, 137 reported at least one episode of combat exposure, and 37 indicated that they were exposed to both sexual assault and combat. Women with combat exposure also described more problems with VHA staff; no other differences were observed for those with and without a combat history. Fontana and colleagues[50] compared different eras of war Veterans by demographics and traumatic exposures. Recent Iraq and Afghanistan serving Veterans differed from Vietnam Veterans by being younger, more often female, more often working, and less often reporting exposure to atrocities in war. Finally, Zouris and colleagues[51] completed a retrospective review of hospitalization data of soldiers evacuated from combat zones in Operation Iraqi Freedom noting most were non-battle injuries (75 percent), Army personnel (83.5 percent) and were male (90 percent). However, ICD-9 diagnoses differed by gender among those wounded or injured with women more often having neoplasms, mental disorders, diseases of the blood, respiratory and genitourinary symptoms compared to the men.

## *Summary of Other Post Trauma Sequelae*

The post-trauma sequelae highlights three visible issues: 1) early TBI data show a preponderance of men from the military; ongoing evaluation is needed to understand what, if any, gender issues may be important for ongoing care; 2) alcohol use in recently returning women Veterans presents greater risk at lower levels of consumption for women with other risk conditions (PTSD MST, combat trauma); and 3) health care utilization by gender and diagnosis requires ongoing follow up because while women may initiate contact with VA sooner, utilization did not differ. Moreover, conditions examined so far for deployed or post-deployed women manifest differently (pain syndromes) or differ in cause for evacuation from theatre. Individual studies also examined a number of other possible associations, such as eating disorders, pain, post-deployment distress, etc.; data are too sparse to draw firm conclusions.

# SUMMARY AND DISCUSSION

## LIMITATIONS

The primary limitation of this review, as with any review, is the possibility that we may have missed relevant articles. We only identified a modest amount of studies. It is possible that there are additional studies which we did not identify. However, our literature search procedures were extensive and included canvassing experts from academia regarding studies we may have missed. It was not possible to conduct formal tests for publication bias, but even with such tests it is not possible to exclude the possibility that such bias exists. Therefore, readers are cautioned about this possibility.

In addition, many of the studies used small sample sizes, or were from single centers or otherwise of questionable generalizability, had poor response rates, and relied on patient self-report for the outcomes of interest, or outcomes of uncertain validity. Therefore, the applicability of conclusions to the general population of deployed women Veterans is uncertain.

## CONCLUSIONS

With the continued expansion of women's role in the military, better understanding of the potential health effects of military service on women during and after their miltary service is essential. While the emerging literature in this area is relatively limited to date, several important themes are nonetheless apparent.

The evidence on the influence of military service on reproductive health is mixed and relies on a modest literature base. Generally, pregnancy outcomes do not appear to differ among deployed vs. undeployed women. However, while several studies demonstrate non-significant differences by deployment status, others present contradictory evidence on the influence of military service on rates of spontaneous abortion, stillbirths, and ectopic pregnancies. Influences on birth outcomes raise more questions than they answer. Only one study reported birthweights, which did not appear to differ by deployment experience of their mothers. More studies have focused on birth defects: about half indicate there are no significant differences in birth defect rates among deployed vs. non-deployed women, whereas the other half report higher rates that are not statistically significant (reflecting problems in statistical power associated with sample sizes for these rare events) or, in fact, reflect higher rates.

The evidence on post-trauma sequellae among OEF/OIF women (soldiers and Veterans) is also relatively limited, and reflects a chief emphasis on mental health issues. Most of these studies are descriptive, and allude to gender differences in diagnosis, impact and health care utilization. Depression and suicide are major foci, demonstrating the highest rates of incident depression among women who are deployed and also exposed to combat. Interestingly, deployment without such exposure was associated with lower rates of incident depression than non-deployment. Women Veterans also had higher risks for depression than men, though lower substance use disorders. Suicide risk was reported as being lower among women Veterans, but the standardized mortality ratio among female Veterans is reportedly higher than that of male Veterans. Several of these studies focused on the differences among Veterans vs. non-Veterans more than women vs. men. For example, the suicide rate among all Veterans (male and female) is estimated to be 66 percent higher than that of the general population. Also, among suicide decedents, women Veterans were 1.6 times more likely to use firearms (compared to non-Veterans).

The literature on mental health needs and utilization among OEF/OIF women Veterans was also descriptive and limited. Younger women Veterans were less likely than young male Veterans to use mental health services, which was in contrast to older Veterans (i.e., older women Veterans were more likely to use mental health services than older male Veterans). This pattern held overall and for those with substance abuse or mood/anxiety disorders, whereas no gender differences were found for PTSD care-seeking. Female soldiers had higher risks of hospitalization for mental disorders, and were more likely to be psychiatric evacuees from the field.

The remainder of the literature on other post-trauma sequelae was variable in topic. The evidence of problem drinking among OEF/OIF women Veterans is mixed (two studies which present contradictory findings). Some of this literature focuses on examing gender differences. For example, predictors of women Veterans' readmission rates for inpatient drug treatment include sexual and physical abuse before, during and after deployment (vs. substance abuse, aggression, and cognitive impairment among men). OEF/OIF women had higher rates of military sexual trauma (MST), and women with MST used VA care more, were less satisfied and had lower perceptions of VA facilities and staff, with particular problems with VA staff among those who had also had combat exposure. OEF/OIF women were less likely to witness the level of killing that men experienced and were less likely to have traumatic brain injuries (TBI) compared to men. Effects of deployment among OEF/OIF women included higher rates of moderate to severe pain, higher distress after the first deployment, and, when added with combat experiences, high rates of eating disorders and extreme weight loss.

## FUTURE RESEARCH

In summary, differential effects of military service by gender are apparent, though the volume and quality of the literature are as yet modest. Given that the published scientific literature not uncommonly reflects prior years' research investment in different topic areas, we anticipate that the investment in women's health research by the U.S. Departments of Veterans Affairs and Defense will contribute to a rapidly growing literature base on the health effects of military service on women over the next several years. Such growth may warrant an updated systematic review, comparable to the overarching review that was recently updated,[4] which demonstrated that more articles were published between 2004 and 2008 than the previous 25 years combined.

More research is needed on the reproductive health effects of military service. Currently, the evidence is mixed with respect to impacts on pregnancy and birth outcomes. One case control study reported an association between rates of birth defects and deployment status, begging the question about what elements of military service (or pursuit of service) might be contributing factors. The available literature also lacks descriptive evidence of the range of reproductive health issues that women in the military and women Veterans face. Currently, there are studies in progress that may well contribute substantively to this knowledge base, but that are not yet in the published literature.

The VA research portfolio on OEF/OIF Veterans' health and health care will also contribute to the emerging literature on the consequences of military service among OEF/OIF women Veterans. The current literature lays some of the groundwork but does so less comprehensively (spanning topics of mental health, physical health, social function, and so on) than would be optimal. Future research should begin to fill these gaps to produce an increasingly detailed portrait of their post-trauma sequelae.

# REFERENCES

1.　　Hazards, O. o. P. H. a. E. Women Veterans Health Care: Facts and Statistics. 2010 [cited 2011; Available from: http://www.publichealth.va.gov/womenshealth/facts.asp.

2.　　Yano, E. M., et al., Toward a VA Women's Health Research Agenda: setting evidence-based priorities to improve the health and health care of women veterans. J Gen Intern Med, 2006. 21 Suppl 3: p. S93-101.

3.　　Goldzweig, C. L., et al., The State of Women Veterans' Health Research. Journal of General Internal Medicine, 2006. 21: p. S82-S92.

4.　　Bean-Mayberry, B., et al., Systematic Review of Women Veterans Health Research 2004-2008, V. HSR&D, Editor. 2010, Evidence Synthesis Program: Washington DC.

5.　　Ngo, A. D., et al., Association between Agent Orange and birth defects: systematic review and meta-analysis. Int J Epidemiol, 2006. 35(5): p. 1220-30.

6.　　Golomb, B. A., Acetylcholinesterase inhibitors and Gulf War illnesses. Proc Natl Acad Sci U S A, 2008. 105(11): p. 4295-300.

7.　　Araneta, M. R., et al., Conception and pregnancy during the Persian Gulf War: the risk to women veterans. Ann Epidemiol, 2004. 14(2): p. 109-16.

8.　　Pierce, P. F., Physical and emotional health of Gulf War veteran women. Aviat Space Environ Med, 1997. 68(4): p. 317-21.

9.　　Kang, H. K., et al., Pregnancy outcomes among U.S. women Vietnam veterans. Am J Ind Med, 2000. 38(4): p. 447-54.

10.　　Kang, H. K., et al., Prevalence of gynecologic cancers among female Vietnam veterans. J Occup Environ Med, 2000. 42(11): p. 1121-7.

11.　　Langlois, P. H., et al., Birth defects and military service since 1990. Mil Med, 2009. 174(2): p. 170-6.

12.　　Araneta, M. R., et al., Birth defects prevalence among infants of Persian Gulf War veterans born in Hawaii, 1989-1993. Teratology, 2000. 62(4): p. 195-204.

13.　　Araneta, M. R., et al., Prevalence of birth defects among infants of Gulf War veterans in Arkansas, Arizona, California, Georgia, Hawaii, and Iowa, 1989-1993. Birth Defects Res A Clin Mol Teratol, 2003. 67(4): p. 246-60.

14.　　Cowan, D. N., et al., The risk of birth defects among children of Persian Gulf War veterans. N Engl J Med, 1997. 336(23): p. 1650-6.

15.　　Gilhooly, P. E., et al., Chronic fatigue and sexual dysfunction in female Gulf War veterans. J Sex Marital Ther, 2001. 27(5): p. 483-7.

16.　　Kang, H., et al., Pregnancy outcomes among U.S. Gulf War veterans: a population-based survey of 30,000 veterans. Ann Epidemiol, 2001. 11(7): p. 504-11.

17.    Murphy, F., et al., Women in the Persian Gulf War: health care implications for active duty troops and veterans. Mil Med, 1997. 162(10): p. 656-60.

18.    Penman, A. D., R. S. Tarver and M. M. Currier, No evidence of increase in birth defects and health problems among children born to Persian Gulf War Veterans in Mississippi. Mil Med, 1996. 161(1): p. 1-6.

19.    Wells, T. S., et al., Self-reported reproductive outcomes among male and female 1991 Gulf War era US military veterans. Matern Child Health J, 2006. 10(6): p. 501-10.

20.    Werler, M. M., J. E. Sheehan and A. A. Mitchell, Gulf War veterans and hemifacial microsomia. Birth Defects Res A Clin Mol Teratol, 2005. 73(1): p. 50-2.

21.    Wittich, A. C., Gynecologic evaluation of the first female soldiers enrolled in the Gulf War Comprehensive Clinical Evaluation Program at Tripler Army Medical Center. Mil Med, 1996. 161(11): p. 635-7.

22.    Zivin, K., et al., Suicide mortality among individuals receiving treatment for depression in the Veterans Affairs health system: associations with patient and treatment setting characteristics. Am J Public Health, 2007. 97(12): p. 2193-8.

23.    Kaplan, M. S., B. H. McFarland and N. Huguet, Firearm suicide among veterans in the general population: findings from the national violent death reporting system. J Trauma, 2009. 67(3): p. 503-7.

24.    McCarthy, J. F., et al., Suicide mortality among patients receiving care in the veterans health administration health system. Am J Epidemiol, 2009. 169(8): p. 1033-8.

25.    Wells, T. S., et al., A prospective study of depression following combat deployment in support of the wars in Iraq and Afghanistan. Am J Public Health, 2010. 100(1): p. 90-9.

26.    Owens, G. P., C. J. Herrera and A. A. Whitesell, A preliminary investigation of mental health needs and barriers to mental health care for female veterans of Iraq and Afghanistan. Traumatology, 2009. 15(2): p. 31-37.

27.    Chatterjee, S., et al., Gender differences in veterans health administration mental health service use: effects of age and psychiatric diagnosis. Womens Health Issues, 2009. 19(3): p. 176-84.

28.    Cohen, B. E., et al., Mental health diagnoses and utilization of VA non-mental health medical services among returning Iraq and Afghanistan veterans. J Gen Intern Med, 2010. 25(1): p. 18-24.

29.    Scott, J. N., Diagnosis and outcome of psychiatric referrals to the Field Mental Health Team, 202 Field Hospital, Op Telic I. J R Army Med Corps, 2005. 151(2): p. 95-100.

30.    Wojcik, B. E., F. Z. Akhtar and L. H. Hassell, Hospital admissions related to mental disorders in U.S. Army soldiers in Iraq and Afghanistan. Mil Med, 2009. 174(10): p. 1010-8.

31.     Rundell, J. R., Demographics of and diagnoses in Operation Enduring Freedom and Operation Iraqi Freedom personnel who were psychiatrically evacuated from the theater of operations. Gen Hosp Psychiatry, 2006. 28(4): p. 352-6.

32.     Seal, K. H., et al., Trends and risk factors for mental health diagnoses among Iraq and Afghanistan veterans using Department of Veterans Affairs health care, 2002–2008. American Journal of Public Health, 2009. 99(9): p. 1651-1658.

33.     Baker, D. G., et al., Trauma exposure, branch of service, and physical injury in relation to mental health among U.S. veterans returning from Iraq and Afghanistan. Mil Med, 2009. 174(8): p. 773-8.

34.     Street, A. E., D. Vogt and L. Dutra, A new generation of women veterans: stressors faced by women deployed to Iraq and Afghanistan. Clin Psychol Rev, 2009. 29(8): p. 685-94.

35.     Seal, K. H., et al., VA mental health services utilization in Iraq and Afghanistan veterans in the first year of receiving new mental health diagnoses. J Trauma Stress, 2010. 23(1): p. 5-16.

36.     LaVela, S. L., et al., Geographical proximity and health care utilization in veterans with SCI&D in the USA. Soc Sci Med, 2004. 59(11): p. 2387-99.

37.     Loney, T. G., The relationship between physical and occupational therapy intensity and rehabilitation outcomes of traumatic brain injury: a comparison of war wounded to non-war wounded persons. TUI University, 2007. 163.

38.     Bell, R. S., et al., Military traumatic brain and spinal column injury: a 5-year study of the impact blast and other military grade weaponry on the central nervous system. J Trauma, 2009. 66(4 Suppl): p. S104-11.

39.     Benda, B., A Study of Substance Abuse, Traumata, and Social Support Systems Among Homeless Veterans. Journal of Human Behavior in the Social Environment Vol 12(1) (2005): 59-82, 2005. 12(q): p. 59-82.

40.     Hawkins, E. J., et al., Recognition and management of alcohol misuse in OEF/OIF and other veterans in the VA: a cross-sectional study. Drug Alcohol Depend, 2010. 109(1-3): p. 147-53.

41.     Nunnink, S. E., et al., Female veterans of the OEF/OIF conflict: concordance of PTSD symptoms and substance misuse. Addict Behav, 2010. 35(7): p. 655-9.

42.     Katz, L. S., et al., Post-Deployment Readjustment Inventory: reliability, validity, and gender differences. Military Psychology, 2010. 22(1): p. 41-56.

43.     Moore, K. R., Predictors of self-reported change in health status among military personnel returning from deployment. Dissertation Abstracts International: Section B: The Sciences and Engineering S2- Dissertation Abstracts International, 2009. 70(3-B): p. 1626.

44.     Fitzgerald, C. E., Improving nurse practitioner assessment of woman veterans. J Am Acad Nurse Pract, 2010. 22(7): p. 339-45.

45.     Adler, A. B., et al., The impact of deployment length and experience on the well-being of male and female soldiers. J Occup Health Psychol, 2005. 10: p. 121-37.

46.     Duggal, M., et al., Comparison of outpatient health care utilization among returning women and men Veterans from Afghanistan and Iraq. BMC Health Serv Res, 2010. 10: p. 175.

47.     Haskell, S. G., et al., Pain among Veterans of Operations Enduring Freedom and Iraqi Freedom: do women and men differ? Pain Med, 2009. 10(7): p. 1167-73.

48.     Jacobson, I. G., et al., Disordered eating and weight changes after deployment: longitudinal assessment of a large US military cohort. Am J Epidemiol, 2009. 169(4): p. 415-27.

49.     Kelly, M. M., et al., Effects of Military Trauma Exposure on Women Veterans' Use and Perceptions of Veteran Health Administration Care. Journal of General Internal Medicine, 2008. 23(6): p. 741-747.

50.     Fontana, A. and R. Rosenheck, Treatment-seeking veterans of Iraq and Afghanistan: comparison with veterans of previous wars. J Nerv Ment Dis, 2008. 196(7): p. 513-21.

51.     Zouris, J. M., A. L. Wade and C. P. Magno, Injury and illness casualty distributions among U.S. Army and Marine Corps personnel during Operation Iraqi Freedom. Mil Med, 2008. 173(3): p. 247-52.

52.     Klausner, A. P., et al., The influence of psychiatric comorbidities and sexual trauma on lower urinary tract symptoms in female veterans. J Urol, 2009. 182(6): p. 2785-90.

53.     LaVela, S., et al., Disease Prevalence and Use of Preventive Services: Comparison of Female Veterans in General and Those with Spinal Cord Injuries and Disorders. MS. Journal of Women's Health, 2006.

54.     Sherman, S. E., et al., Gender differences in smoking cessation services received among veterans. Womens Health Issues, 2005. 15(3): p. 126-33.

55.     Stecker, T., et al., Characteristics of women seeking intensive outpatient substance use treatment in the VA. J Womens Health (Larchmt), 2007. 16(10): p. 1478-84.

# APPENDIX 1. SEARCH STRATEGIES

## REPRODUCTIVE (8/4/2010)

**DATABASE SEARCHED & TIME PERIOD COVERED:**
  PubMed – 1966-8/4/2010

**LANGUAGE:**
  English

**SEARCH STRATEGY:**
reproductive OR reproduction OR pregnan* OR birth* OR fertility OR infertility OR infertile
OR menstrual OR menstruation OR menses OR urinary tract OR sexually transmitted OR hiv
OR cervical OR ovarian OR genital OR gynecologic* OR "Congenital Abnormalities"[Mesh]
AND
veteran*[tiab] OR veteran*[mh] OR military personnel
AND
female* OR women* OR woman OR gender OR women's health

=================================================

## OEF/OIF (8/2/2010)

**DATABASE SEARCHED & TIME PERIOD COVERED:**
  PubMed – 1990-8/2/2010

**LANGUAGE:**
  English

**SEARCH STRATEGY:**
veteran*[tiab] OR veteran*[mh] OR military personnel
AND
female* OR women* OR woman OR gender OR women's health
AND
gulf war OR persian gulf OR "desert storm" OR iraq* OR afghanistan OR OEF OR OIF OR
"enduring freedom" OR afghan

=====================================================================

**DATABASE SEARCHED & TIME PERIOD COVERED:**
  PsycINFO – 1990-8/2/2010

**LANGUAGE:**
  English

**SEARCH STRATEGY:**
veteran* OR military personnel
AND
 female* OR women* OR woman OR gender

AND

gulf war OR persian gulf OR "desert storm" OR iraq* OR afghanistan OR OEF OR OIF OR "enduring freedom" OR afghan

Population Group: Female
Search modes - Phrase Searching (Boolean)

===========================================================

**DATABASE SEARCHED & TIME PERIOD COVERED:**
 CINAHL (Cumulative Index to Nursing & Allied Health Literature) – 1990-8/2/2010

**LANGUAGE:**
 English

**SEARCH STRATEGY:**
veteran* OR military personnel
AND
female* OR women* OR woman OR gender
AND
gulf war OR persian gulf OR "desert storm" OR iraq* OR afghanistan OR OEF OR OIF OR "enduring freedom" OR afghan

Gender: Female
Search modes - Phrase Searching (Boolean)

===========================================================

**DATABASE SEARCHED & TIME PERIOD COVERED:**
 Social Science Abstracts – 1990-8/2/2010

**LANGUAGE:**
 English

**SEARCH STRATEGY:**
veteran* OR military personnel
AND
female* OR women* OR woman OR gender
AND
gulf war OR persian gulf OR "desert storm" OR iraq* OR afghanistan OR OEF OR OIF OR "enduring freedom" OR afghan

Search modes - Phrase Searching (Boolean)

# APPENDIX 2. KEY QUESTION #1 EVIDENCE TABLE

| Author | Sample Characteristics | Sample Size | Design/Objective | Main Measures | Main Findings |
|---|---|---|---|---|---|
| Araneta; 2000[12] | Infants born to Gulf War Veterans (GWV) non-deployed Veterans (NDV) who were registered in Hawaii Birth Defects Program in 1989-1993. | 17,187 military infants of GWV and NDV in Hawaii were identified. | Compare prevalence of selected congenital anomalies between:<br>1. GWV and NDV conceived before the war<br>2. GWV and NDV conceived during or after war<br>3. Prewar/postwar conceptions of GWV population-based study | 48 major birth defects prevalence among military births in Hawaii through the first year of life | Prevalence of 48 selected birth defects was similar in NDV and GWV groups in conceptions that happened before the war and conceptions during and after the Gulf war.<br><br>Among GWV infants, the prevalence of 48 selected birth defects did not differ among prewar and postwar conceptions.<br><br>Limitations: small numbers of case infants with birth defects- not enough statistical power for rare birth defects.<br><br>Unable to evaluate role of maternal GWV exposure because small numbers of births in female GWV (165 births) in Hawaii. |
| Araneta; 2003[7] | Deployment data and inpatient records from military hospitals. | 1,558 females | Compare reproductive outcomes of Gulf War with postwar conceptions of women deployed and non-deployed. | Adverse reproductive outcomes, spontaneous abortions, ectopic pregnancies | Gulf War exposed conceptions and non-deployed conceptions had similar outcomes. However, Gulf War Veterans postwar conceptions were at increased risk of ectopic pregnancies and spontaneous abortions. |
| Araneta; 2003[13] | Infants born to Gulf War Veterans (GWV) non-deployed Veterans (NDV) who were registered in Arkansas, Arizona, California, Georgia, Hawaii and Iowa Birth Defects Program, a population-based birth defect registries, in 1989-1993 | 11,961 military infants of GWV and 33,052 military infants of NDV registered in Arkansas, Arizona, California, Georgia, Hawaii and Iowa were identified. | Determine prevalence of selected congenital anomalies between:<br>1. GWV and NDV conceived before the war<br>2. GWV and NDV conceived during or after war<br>3. Prewar/postwar conceptions of GWV population-based study | 48 major birth defects prevalence among military births in Hawaii through the first year of life | Higher prevalence of tricuspid valve insufficiency, aortic valve stenosis, and renal agenesis or hypoplasia in infants conceived to post war GWV men.<br><br>Higher prevalence of hypospadias in infants conceived postwar to female GWV.<br><br>Above persisted after adjustment for known risk factors and population differences.<br><br>No difference in risk for any of combined 48 selected defects by deployment status. |

**Health Effects of Military Service on Women Veterans**

| Author | Sample Characteristics | Sample Size | Design/Objective | Main Measures | Main Findings |
|---|---|---|---|---|---|
| Cowan; 1997[14] | Live births at 135 military hospitals 1991-1993 | GWV offspring<br><br>• 30.151 live births born to 29,468 male GWV<br><br>• 32,638 live births born to 31,646 male NDV<br><br>• 3,847 live births to 3722 women GWV<br><br>• 8,825 live births to 8494 women NDVW | To compare overall risk of birth defects among offspring of GWV to offspring of non deployed Veterans (NDV) | Occurrence of birth defects noted in the medical file. ICD-9-CM code related to congenital malformations | • No increase in birth defects among children of GWV.<br>• Prevalence of any birth defect was 7.45% for deployed Veterans and 7.59% for non-deployed Veterans (RR 0.98, 95% CI 0.93-1.03).<br>• No significant association between service in the Gulf War and prevalence of any birth defect for male Veterans (OR 0.97, 95% CI 0.91-1.03) or female Veterans (OR 1.07, 95% CI 0.94-1.22).<br>• The unadjusted OR for having an infant with severe birth defects was 1.03 (95% CI 0.92-1.15) for male active-duty Veterans, 0.92 (95% CI 0.71-1.20) for female active duty Veterans, and 1.00 (95% CI 0.90-1.10) for men and women combined.<br>• Limitation: military facilities only. |
| Gilhooly; 2001[15] | Previously deployed female US Persian Gulf Veterans enrolled in New Jersey Persian Gulf War Research Center Study | 46 Female | Relationship between sexual dysfunction in female Gulf War Veterans | This study evaluated sexual dysfunction in Veterans with and without chronic fatigue. | Chronic fatigue is one of the most chronic conditions reported by Gulf War Veterans. Includes 22 healthy subjects and 26 with fatigue. Female sexual dysfunction was reported by 10% of control and by 60% of those with fatigue (p value < .002). 19% vs 81% (p value < .001) decrease in libido. |
| Kang; 2000[9] | U.S. women Veterans in the U.S. military during the period July 4, 1965 through March 28, 1973 | 8,280 US women Veterans (4140 deployed, 4140 not deployed) | Comparison of self-reported pregnancy outcomes among women Veterans who were deployed to Vietnam and those who were not | Risk of having children with moderate to severe birth defects was significantly elevated among Vietnam Veterans. | The risk of birth defects among index children was significantly associated with mother's military service in Vietnam. |
| Kang; 2000[10] | U.S. women Veterans in the U.S. military during the period July 4, 1965 through March 28, 1973 | 4,140 Female | Structured telephone interview including history of gynecologic cancer | The association between the risk of GYN cancer and military service in Vietnam | Female Vietnam Veterans did not experience a higher prevalence of GYN cancer in the 30 years since the conflict. |
| Kang; 2001[16] | Gulf War Veterans | 11,441 Gulf War Veterans and 9476 control subjects | Comparison of reproductive outcomes among US Gulf War Veterans and non-Gulf War Veterans | Miscarriages and birth defects | This survey suggests that female Gulf War Veterans report significantly higher rates of birth defects than do military control subjects. |

**Health Effects of Military Service on Women Veterans**

| Author | Sample Characteristics | Sample Size | Design/Objective | Main Measures | Main Findings |
|---|---|---|---|---|---|
| Langlois; 2009[11] | Population based Case control study – National Birth Defects Prevention Study (NBDPS) | Cases born Oct 1999 to Dec 2003. 150 cases and 3 exposed cases | Population based Case control study– National Birth Defects Prevention Study (NBDPS) | Association between cohorts and active duty birth over 30 major defects | • No statistically significant associations between maternal or paternal military service and elevated risk of selected birth defects.<br><br>• Of the 35 birth defects presented, 5 exhibited adjusted odds ratios above 1.50: hydrocephalus, atrioventricular septal defects, anomalous pulmonary venous return, heterotaxia, and omphalocele – though not statistically significant.<br><br>⇨ None of the odds ratios 1.00 were statistically significant.<br><br>• Tricuspid atresia exhibited the highest crude odds ratio (2.03), but that decreased to 1.43 after adjustment for maternal age, race/ethnicity, and education. |
| Murphy; 1997[17] | Female troops deployed to the Persian Gulf | 10,00 Female and 15,000 Male | Literature review and analysis of VA and DoD health registries to determine healthcare use and needs of female Veterans | Diagnoses and symptoms by gender | This article found female health care needs to be similar to those of their male counterparts, with the exception of gynecologic issues. More data is needed, especially for determining long-term health care needs after deployment. |
| Penman; 1996[18] | Population based registries used to determine Live born and Stillborn children born after deployment to National Guard personnel in two units in southeast Mississippi from Dec 1993-May 1994 | 54 children<br><br>6 mothers were Veterans (including one family with both parents Veterans) | Data reviewed from 2 population based registries<br><br>1. Metropolitan Atlanta Congenital Defects Program<br>2. Centers for Disease Controls' Birth Defects Monitoring Program California Birth Defects Monitoring Program | Birth Defects<br><br>Still Births<br><br>Deaths | • The observed number of birth defects among was not greater than expected on the basis of population-based registries.<br><br>• 3 cases of major birth defects, 2 cases of minor birth defects, No stillbirths, no deaths. |

**Health Effects of Military Service on Women Veterans**

| Author | Sample Characteristics | Sample Size | Design/Objective | Main Measures | Main Findings |
|---|---|---|---|---|---|
| Pierce; 1997[8] | Female Veterans post Gulf War from the DoD Manpower Data Center | 525 Female | Conducted a survey to collect demographic data, as well as physical and mental health data | Multiple statistical analyses were used to describe women's physical/ emotional health the two times point following the GW. | 525 women participated in the study following the war and again in a follow up study two years later (sampled from members of the Air Force: active, guard, or reserve). Measures included general physical health, gender specific health, "Gulf War Syndrome," and PTSD. Multiple statistical analyses were used to describe women's physical and emotional health at two time points following the war. Deployed female Veterans reported significantly more general and gender specific health problems than did women who were not deployed in that conflict. Findings from this study suggest the need for further study concerning gynecological and reproductive health. |
| Wells; 2006[19] | Deployed and non-deployed Gulf War era Veterans | 2,233 female, 2,159 male participants | Comparison of deployed and non-deployed Veterans surveyed on self-reported reproductive outcomes | Reproductive outcomes (birth weight, number of pregnancies)  Adverse reproductive outcomes (ectopic pregnancies, stillbirths, miscarriages) | • No difference in number of pregnancies, birth weight of infants.  • Neither gender of deployed Gulf War Veterans significantly differed from non-deployed Veterans in adverse reproductive outcomes. |
| Werler; 2004[20] | Cases from craniofacial clinics in 26 cities (US and Canada) and matched to 832 controls by pediatrician and child's age  HFM cases ≤ 3 years old (born 1996-2002) | Birth year of cases to controls were 1996-2002. There were 232 cases and 832 controls.  Four mothers and 30 fathers served in the military, and 10 control mothers and 100 control fathers also served in the military | Retrospective Case-control study  Describe relationship between Hemifacial microsomia HFM) (Goldenhar syndrome) risk and parental military service (including Gulf War) | Measure Gulf War Service that occurred between 5 and 11 years before pregnancy  Odds ratio of risk of multi adjusted odds ratio of HFM in those serving in the Gulf war for five to 11 years before pregnancy. Association of gulf or military service with HFM | • Mothers of 4 cases and 10 controls reported military service before and after pregnancy.  • Neither military service overall or Gulf War Service was associated with HFM risk. Odds ratio for any parental military service was elevated- but not statistically significant.  • Parental army service assoc with 2.4 fold increase of HFM- after adjusting for race, income, twin, and low body mass. (OR 2.4, 95% CI 1.4-4.2), parental GW army service (OR 2.8, 95% CI 0.8-9.6);  • Association with any parent served in the Gulf War was not increased (OR 0.8, 95% CI 0.3-2.3). |
| Wittich; 1996[21] | Women enrolled in DoD Persian Gulf Illness Comprehensive Clinical Evaluation Program at Tripler Army Medical Center | 17 females, 16 served in Gulf War and 1 dependent of Gulf War Veteran | Description of the sample's treatments during the program and reproductive histories | N/A | Services and histories are described, with 8 Veterans experiencing gynecologic problems while serving in the Gulf, and 43% since returning in 1991. Six patients became pregnant after returning, with 1 patient suffering miscarriages. |

# APPENDIX 3. KEY QUESTION 2 EVIDENCE TABLE

| Author | Sample Characteristics | Sample Size | Design/Objective | Main Measures | Main Findings |
|---|---|---|---|---|---|
| Adler; 2005[45] | U.S. female and male soldiers in non-combat arms units deployed on a NATO peacekeeping mission to the Bosnia area of operations that included Hungary, Bosnia-Herzegovina, and Croatia | Females 1,225 Males 2,114 | Observational; To examine the effects of stressor duration (deployment length) and stressor novelty (no prior deployment experience) on the psychological health of male and female military personnel returning from a peacekeeping deployment | Correlations between demographics, deployment experience, and dependent variables by gender; length of deployment and mean scale score of depressive and posttraumatic stress symptoms by gender; deployment experience and mean scale score of depressive and posttraumatic stress symptoms by gender | Longer deployments and 1st-time deployments were associated with an increase in distress scores. However, the relationship between deployment length and increased distress was found only for male soldiers. |
| Baker; 2009[33] | Newly registered OEF/OIF Veterans and reservists, who consecutively enrolled for general care in the VA San Diego Healthcare System and completed a battery of questionnaires between April and October 2006 | 339 | Observational; To more comprehensively characterize the OEF/OIF mental health concerns, examining the relationship between demographic factors, military service characteristics, combat-related injury, and mental health symptoms | Demographic and military service-related characteristics, mental health caseness, predictors of PTSD | • A minority (36%) did not screen positive for mental health symptoms; the remainder met threshold for caseness of PTSD, depression, or substance and alcohol abuse.<br><br>• Using a hierarchical logistic regression model, gender, age, race, and rank were not significantly related to PTSD caseness, whereas most recent branch of service and report of injury during combat were.<br><br>• Follow-up analyses revealed that trauma history and combat exposure varied by branch of service. |
| Bell; 2009[38] | Inpatient admissions to 2 military hospitals over a 5 year period from a closed or penetrating head trauma suffered during combat operations in Iraq | Females 7 Males 401 | Observational; To describe a military hospital experience with severe closed and penetrating central nervous system trauma associated with conventional and unconventional warfare | Primary measures include type of injury, mechanisms, initial Glasgow coma scale (GCS), discharge GCS score, admission injury severity score (ISS), total intensive care unit (ICU) days, Glasgow Outcome Scale scores at discharge, 6 months, and 1-2 years | Most head injuries were male (98%), and most sustained penetrating brain injury with explosive blast accounting for the predominant mechanism of injury. The presence of CSF leak, vascular injury, and penetrating trauma resulted in higher ISS levels and ICU stays. (No gender specific results are reported.) |

**Health Effects of Military Service on Women Veterans**

| Author | Sample Characteristics | Sample Size | Design/Objective | Main Measures | Main Findings |
|---|---|---|---|---|---|
| Benda; 2005[39] | Convenience sample of all homeless female Veterans that entered an inpatient VA domiciliary program for substance abuse in a 3-year period. Systematic random sample of homeless men that entered program during same period. | Females 310 Males 315 | Observational; (1) to study gender differences in predictors of readmission to inpatient drug treatment among homeless Veterans because VA medical centers currently do not have services that are designed specifically for women; (2) are abuses at different stages of life span, combat exposure, and recent traumatic events commensurate predictors; do employment, housing, family or friend relationships and spirituality mediate (3) or moderate (4) relationships between trauma and relapse. | Re-admission to inpatient drug treatment in a two-year follow-up | Sexual and physical abuse in childhood or during active duty in the military and during the past 2 years were most potent predictors of readmission for women than men. Women's readmission was heightened by increases in depression, suicidal thoughts, and traumatic events. Women's readmission was lessened by greater family, friend, church or other support.<br><br>-Men's readmission increased with greater substance abuse, aggression, and cognitive impairment. Men's readmission decreases with employment stability and job satisfaction. |
| Chatterjee; 2009[27] | National sample of Veterans with at least 1 outpatient visit in the VHA in FY99 associated with a mental health or substance abuse (SA) diagnosis | 782,789 | Observational; To compare gender differences in mental health disease burden and outpatient mental health utilization among Veterans utilizing Veterans Health Administration (VHA) mental health services | Odds of utilizing mental health and specialty mental health services by gender, age, and diagnostic category | • Younger women Veterans (<35 years old) were significantly less likely and older women (≥35) more likely to use any mental health services in comparison with their male counterparts.<br>• Similar findings were observed for younger women diagnosed with SA or mood and anxiety disorders, but not among Veterans with PTSD or bipolar and psychotic disorders, among whom there were no gender or age differences.<br>• In the case of specialized services for SA or PTSD, women younger than 55 with SA or PTSD were significantly less likely to use services than men.<br>• Women Veterans underutilized specialty mental health services in relation to men but receipt of mental health care overall in FY99 varied by age and diagnosis. |

**Health Effects of Military Service on Women Veterans**

| Author | Sample Characteristics | Sample Size | Design/Objective | Main Measures | Main Findings |
|---|---|---|---|---|---|
| Cohen; 2009[28] | National sample of Veterans newly utilizing VA healthcare between October 7, 2001 and March 31, 2007, followed until March 31, 2008 | 249,440 | Observational; To compare utilization across three groups of Iraq and Afghanistan Veterans: those without mental disorders, those with mental disorders other than PTSD, and those with PTSD | Variations in utilization of VA non-mental health services by mental health diagnoses | • Veterans with mental disorders had 42-146% greater utilization than those without mental disorders, depending on the service category (all p<0.001).<br><br>• Those with PTSD had the highest utilization in all categories: 71-170% greater utilization than those without mental disorders (all p< 0.001).<br><br>• In adjusted analyses, compared with Veterans without mental disorders, those with mental disorders other than PTSD had 55% higher utilization of all non-mental health outpatient services; those with PTSD had 91% higher utilization.<br><br>• Female sex and lower rank were also independently associated with greater utilization. |
| Duggal; 2010[46] | Sample of female and male Operation Enduring Freedom (OEF) and Operation Iraqi Freedom (OIF) Veterans seeking healthcare services in the VA system | Females 240<br>Males 1,380 | Observational; To examine gender differences in the utilization of VA outpatient health care services | Outpatient VA service use included basic care (e.g., primary care, mental health, or specialty care). Initiation of care was defined as one visit or more to outpatient care after return from deployment and intensity of utilization was defined as the total number of outpatient visits during the study period. | Women were more likely to be younger, single, and non-white compared to men. Women were more likely to use outpatient care services (OR 1.47, 95% CI 1.09, 1.98), but once initiated, frequency of visits over time did not differ by gender (incident rate ratio [IRR] 1.07, 95% CI 0.90, 1.27). |
| Fitzgerald; 2010[44] | Clinical guide to use screening tools for post traumatic stress disorder, traumatic brain injury, and military sexual trauma in the civilian setting | N/A | Clinical Practice Guideline;<br>To provide nurse practitioners with a brief screening tools to be used during routine office visits to assist with accurate identification of post military health concerns | Not applicable | Potential benefits include more effective and comprehensive care to a growing female population with a history of military service seen for routine care. Brief screening instruments can help providers formulate accurate diagnoses of service related conditions with appropriate treatment and referral. |

**Health Effects of Military Service on Women Veterans**

| Author | Sample Characteristics | Sample Size | Design/Objective | Main Measures | Main Findings |
|---|---|---|---|---|---|
| Fontana; 2008[50] | Administrative sample of female and male Veterans in VA Northeast Program of Evaluation Center (NEPEC) database who sought treatment from a VA specialized program for PTSD and served in a war zone during only 1 of 3 recent wars | Total 36,413 (Sex not specified) | Observational; To compare current Iraq/Afghanistan Veterans with 4 samples of outpatient and inpatient Persian Gulf and Vietnam Veterans | Socio-demographic characteristics, traumatic exposures (i.e., receiving hostile/friendly fire, participating in atrocities, and witnessing atrocities without participating), and clinical status including | Recent Iraq/Afghanistan Veterans differed most notably from Vietnam Veterans by being younger, more likely to be female, less likely to be married or separated/divorced, more often working, less likely to report exposure to atrocities in military. Iraq/Afghanistan Veterans less often diagnosed with substance abuse disorders, manifested more violent behaviors, and had lower rates of VA disability compensation because of PTSD. |
| Haskell; 2009[47] | National sample of Veterans from OEF/OIF roster from Defense Manpower Data Center containing all personnel discharged from US Military between October 1, 2001 to November 30, 2007 who enrolled for VA services or received VA care before January 1, 2008 | Females 18,481 Males 134,731 | Observational; To evaluate sex differences in the prevalence, severity, and persistence of pain among OEF/OIF Veterans seen at VA outpatient clinic visits during the year after returning from deployment | Measures included pain numeric rating scores recorded at all outpatient visits, defined moderate to severe pain as >/= 4 rating, persistent pain defined as 3 or more pain scores >/= 4 recorded in at least 3 different months, ICD-9 codes for diagnoses of PTSD or depression if codes occurred on two or more outpatient visits, and demographic data | No significant difference was present for the probability of pain assessment by sex in bivariate and regression analysis (RR 0.98, 95%CI 0.96, 1.00). Female Veterans were less likely to report any pain compared to male (RR 0.89, 95%CI 0.86, 0.92). Among those with pain, female Veterans were more likely to report moderate-severe pain (RR 1.05, 95%CI 1.01, 1.09) and less likely to have persistent pain (RR 0.90, 95%CI 0.81, 0.99). When stratified by diagnosis, Veterans with depression or PTSD were more likely to be assessed for pain (p<.0001). However, there was no significant difference in the proportion of Veterans assessed for pain by sex in those with PTSD and depression (p>.05 in both cases). |
| Hawkins; 2010[40] | National sample of Veterans in VA screened for alcohol use between October 1, 2006, and September 30, 2007, and under age 55 | Females 2,009 Males 10,083 | Observational; To evaluate the recognition and management of alcohol misuse in OEF/OIF Veterans enrolled in the VA system | Alcohol Use Disorders Identification Test Consumptions questions (AUDIT-C 10 question); military service information; documentation of brief intervention, referral, and completed referral for treatment | Age-specific and total prevalence of alcohol misused was higher for younger OEF/OIF men vs. non OEF/OIF men. Rates of alcohol misuse were lower in both OEF/OIF and non OEF/OIF women. No significant difference was observed in the prevalence of alcohol misuse between OEF/OIF and non OEF/OIF women. |
| Jacobson; 2009[48] | Population based sample of randomly selected military service members on rosters as of October 2000 from Millennium Cohort Study | Total 42,174 (Sex not specified) | Observational; To investigate disordered eating levels before and after deployment to determine the prospective association between stressful life events and the development of eating disorders | Disordered eating from 8 question survey from the Patient Health Questionnaire, weight change from baseline to follow up by self-report, demographics and military data | Women deployed with combat exposures were 1.78 times more likely to develop disordered eating (95%CI 1.02, 3.11) and 2.35 times more likely to lose an extreme amount of weight (95%CI 1.17, 4.70). |

**Health Effects of Military Service on Women Veterans**

| Author | Sample Characteristics | Sample Size | Design/Objective | Main Measures | Main Findings |
|---|---|---|---|---|---|
| Kaplan; 2009[23] | Suicide decedents aged 18 years and older from the combined 2003 to 2006 National Violent Death Reporting System | 28,534 | Observational; To examine the rate, prevalence, and relative odds of firearm use among Veteran suicide decedents in the general population | Total and firearm specific suicide rates by gender, Veteran status, and age groups | • Across the age groups, male and female Veterans had higher firearm suicide rates than non-Veterans.<br><br>• Among males and females, younger Veterans (18-34 years) had the highest firearm and total suicide rates.<br><br>• The male and female Veteran suicide decedents were, respectively, 1.3 and 1.6 times more likely to use firearms relative to non-Veterans after adjusting for age, marital status, race, and region of residence.<br><br>• Although violent death and use of firearms are generally associated with men, the results reported here suggest that firearms among female Veterans deserve particular attention among health professional within and outside the Veterans Affairs system. |
| Katz; 2010[42] | Sample of post-deployed service members from OEF/OIF duty | Females 32<br>Males 183 | Observational; To gather psychometric information on the newly developed Post-Deployment Readjustment Inventory (PDRI); validity testing | PDRI global scale and 6 subscales, General information form, Brief Symptom Inventory (BSI), Posttraumatic Checklist-Military version (PCL-M), demographics, and 5 items assessing exposure to war stressors: MST; being injured; and witnessing others injured or killed | The PDRI was highly correlated with the BSI, the PCL-M, and the items for substance abuse. Exposure to war events, scores of readjustment and symptoms were compared across gender. Overall MANOVA was not significant. However, they differed on type of exposure. Women reported a higher rate of MST than men, and men reported higher rate of witnessing others injured or killed than women. |
| Kelly; 2008[49] | National, cross-sectional sample of female Veterans from the National Registry of Women Veterans stratified by age group, period of service, and race (black and non-black) | Females 1,496 | Observational; To investigate the effects of military sexual assault and combat exposure on women Veterans' use of Veterans Health Administration (VHA) services and perceptions of VHA care. | Military sexual assault history, combat exposure, use of VHA services, satisfaction with VHA services | Women Veterans with histories of military sexual assault reported more use of VHA services, but less satisfaction, poorer perceptions of VHA facilities and staff, and more problems with VHA services compared to women Veterans without histories of sexual assault. Combat exposure was related to more problems with VHA staff, although few other differences were observed for women with and without histories of combat exposure. |

| Author | Sample Characteristics | Sample Size | Design/Objective | Main Measures | Main Findings |
|---|---|---|---|---|---|
| Klausner; 2009[52] | Sample of women referred to a specialized lower urinary tract symptom clinic compared to women in a primary care clinic in a VA medical center | Females 1,298 | Observational; To characterize the association of psychiatric co-morbidities and sexual trauma with lower urinary tract symptoms (LUTS) | Survey items completed included the Incontinence Impact Questionnaire-7 to assess quality of life and Urogenital Distress Inventory -6 to assess symptoms, sexual trauma screening, pregnancy and birth histories, and psychiatric co-morbidities. | Women referred for LUTS evaluations had higher rates of psychiatric co-morbidities (64.5% vs. 25.9%, p<.001) and sexual trauma (49.6% vs. 20.1%, p<.001) compared to women in primary care. Stepwise multivariate regression demonstrated that higher UDI-6 scores associated with age<50 and history of miscarriage, while higher IIG-7 scores associated with psychiatric co-morbidities and history of miscarriage. |
| LaVela; 2006[53] | Female Veteran data from a national cross-sectional survey mailed to Paralyzed Veterans of America (PVA) members for the SCI&D group and data from the CDC 2003 Behavioral Risk Factor Surveillance System (BRFSS) survey for the non-SCI&D comparison group | Females 593 | Observational; To compare disease prevalence and preventive service use among female Veterans in general and those with spinal cord injuries and disorders (SCI&D) | Disease/condition prevalence (asthma, diabetes, myocardial infarction, stroke, coronary heart disease, high blood pressure, high cholesterol, tooth decay/gum disease, injuries), health status (general health, physical and mental health), and use of preventive services (cholesterol check, dental care, influenza and pneumonia vaccinations, colon screening, breast and cervical cancer screening) among women Veterans with and without SCI&D | Female Veterans with SCI&D were similar in age and race but were better educated and less likely to be employed than female Veterans in general. Coronary heart disease (CHD) prevalence was higher in those with SCI&D (17% vs. 8%, p < 0.0001). Health status was lower in SCI&D (27%) than in general female Veterans (41%), p = 0.002. Fewer women with SCI&D, than female Veterans in general reported having received recommended dental care (56% vs. 69%, p=0.004), colon screening in prior 5 years (59% vs. 72%, p = 0.023) or prior 10 years (67% vs. 92%, p < 0.0001), mammogram (84% vs. 91%, p = 0.019), and Pap smear (88% vs. 98%, p < 0.0001). There were no differences in receipt of respiratory vaccinations or cholesterol screening. |

**Health Effects of Military Service on Women Veterans**

| Author | Sample Characteristics | Sample Size | Design/Objective | Main Measures | Main Findings |
|---|---|---|---|---|---|
| LaVela; 2004[36] | Veterans with spinal cord injuries and disorders (SCI&D) identified with the Spinal Cord Dysfunction Registry (SCD-R) for 2001 | Total 8,983 98% male | Observational; To describe inpatient and outpatient health care utilization of Veterans with SCI&D; to determine whether health care utilization patterns differ based on residing longer or shorter distances from sources of care; to determine if VA facility closest to patient is bypassed in order to receive care at another VA facility | Utilization defined as any inpatient or outpatient health care services, history of illness (defined as 1 hospitalization in the prior year), travel distance between the zip code center to the VA facility used, and travel distance to the nearest VA | Patients used OP services less frequently when VA facilities were farther away from their residences. Male Veterans with SCI&D were less likely than females Veterans to utilize OP care ($p < .0000$). Being male reduced the number of OP visits by 27%. |
| Loney; 2007[37] | Sample of soldiers with traumatic brain injury (war wounded and non war wounded) admitted to one VA medical center for physical and occupational therapy between January 1, 2004 and December 31, 2005 | Females 10 Males 109 | Dissertation/ Observational; To identify which variables are most associated with therapy intensity and functional clinical outcomes in war wounded traumatic brain injury soldiers from OEF/OIF | Therapy intensity was measured in terms of duration, functional independent measure (FIM), FIM change and FIM efficiency, Severity of injury and TBI polytrauma/blast co-morbidities | War wounded TBI patients had lower admission FIM scores ($M = 77.09$, $SD = 41.55$), admission Mobility FIM scores ($M = 21.66$, $SD = 12.85$) and spent longer time between initial injury and admission to rehabilitation ($M = 92.81$, $SD = 110.80$) than the non-war wounded admission FIM scores ($M = 68.18$, $SD = 32.23$), admission Mobility FIM scores ($M = 19.00$, $SD = 10.78$), and shorter time between initial injury and admission to rehabilitation ($M = 57.58$, $SD = 63.91$). (No specific findings were given by gender. Gender was used in models.) |

**Health Effects of Military Service on Women Veterans**

| Author | Sample Characteristics | Sample Size | Design/Objective | Main Measures | Main Findings |
|---|---|---|---|---|---|
| McCarthy; 2009[24] | All Veterans with inpatient or outpatient services utilization in any VHA facility during fiscal year 2000 or fiscal year 2001 using data from the VHA's National Patient Care Database | 4,670,968 | Observational; To examine suicide rates among VHA patients and compare them with rates in general population | Mortality ratios for suicide risks among VHA patients for age and gender subgroups compared with those in the general US population | • Overall, for men and women combined, suicide risks among VHA patients were 66% higher than those observed in the general US population.<br>• VHA rates were 43.13/100,000 person-years for men and 10.41/100,000 person-years for women.<br>• For male patients, the age-adjusted standardized mortality ratio was 1.66; for females, it was 1.87.<br>• Male patients aged 30-79 years had increased risks relative to men in the general population; standardized mortality ratios ranged from 2.56 (ages 30-39 years) to 1.33 (ages 70-79 years).<br>• Female patients aged 40-59 years had greater risks than did women in the general population, with standardized mortality ratios of 2.15 (ages 40-49) and 2.36 (ages 50-5 years). |
| Moore; 2009[43] | Cohort of service members who repeated their PDHA from deployments to OIF/OEF in 2004-2005 | Females 1,061 Males 7,777 | Dissertation/ Observational; To identify the health concerns and symptoms that changed, during and after deployment and predicted repeat PDHA | Post Deployment Health Assessment (PDHA), and demographics | Results yielded significant values for age, gender, service, and length of deployment with changes in health concerns. Females were less likely than males to report health changes (OR 0.542, 95%CI 0.470, 0.626). There was a significant correlation between service members that were female (r=.26, p=.013); had shorter deployments (r=-.050, p=.000); and were older (r=.28, p=.009) for increased changes in their second PDHA. Change in health symptoms occurred for 12 of 19 symptoms measured. |
| Nunnink; 2010[41] | Newly enrolling female Veterans in 1 southern California VA Medical Center | Females 36 | Observational; To examine the rates of co-morbid PTSD and substance abuse in an all-female OEF/ OIF Veteran sample, and to investigate the differences in substance abuse in women screening positive vs. screening negative for PTSD | Alcohol Use Disorders Identification Test (AUDIT 10) for alcohol screening, Drug Abuse Screening Test (DAST), the Davidson Trauma Scale (DTS) to measure PTSD symptomatology, demographics, discharge type, and screening items for exposure to combat and problems with alcohol | Thirty-one percent (11) of this small sample of OEF/ OIF female Veterans screened positive for PTSD symptoms, 47% (17) screened positive for high-risk drinking and 6% (2) screened positive for drug abuse. Alcohol and drug misuse were both good predictors of PTSD symptoms. Increase awareness and screening for both PTSD and alcohol problems in female Veterans is paramount. |

**Health Effects of Military Service on Women Veterans**

| Author | Sample Characteristics | Sample Size | Design/Objective | Main Measures | Main Findings |
|---|---|---|---|---|---|
| Owens; 2009[26] | Female Veterans of Iraq and Afghanistan who completed an online survey for the study | 50 | Observational; To examine the mental health needs and barriers to mental health service use specifically for female Veterans of the wars in Iraq and Afghanistan | Combat exposure and mental health symptoms, mental health services utilization, comparisons between treatment seeker and non-treatment seekers, barriers to seeking mental health services in the VA system | • The most frequently reported concerns for which participants indicated they needed counseling were depression, relationship issues, anxiety, and anger management.<br>• Although 78% of respondents reported that they felt they needed treatment in the past year, 42% of these individuals indicated that they did not seek counseling.<br>• Two commonly reported barriers to seeking mental health services in the VA were long waiting periods for appointments and prior bad experiences.<br>• Mental health concerns and symptoms of returning female Veterans indicate the need for treatment, but a significant gap remains in the self-reported need for assistance and seeking of services. |
| Rundell; 2006[31] | Records of consecutive OEF/OIF patients who were medially evacuated to the Landstuhl Regional Medical Center (LRMC) in Germany from the theater of operations for primarily psychiatric reasons between November 4, 2001, and July 30, 2004 | 1,264 | Descriptive; To characterize the demographic and clinical information of OEF and OIF military personnel who were psychiatrically evacuated from the theater of operations | Demographic and administrative characteristics, psychiatric diagnoses | • When compared with all returned OEF/OIF Veterans, psychiatric evacuees were more likely to be: female, under the age of 31 years, African-American or Hispanic, enlisted and National Guard/Reserve.<br>• Over 80% of patients were evacuated during the first 6 months, compared with 17% during the second 6 months of deployment.<br>• The most common diagnostic categories were adjustment disorders (37.6%), mood disorders (22.1%), personality disorders (15.7%) and anxiety disorders (15.4%); 16.5 % received no psychiatric diagnosis.<br>• Only 5% of evacuees returned to OEF/OIF duty.<br>• Almost half of evacuated patients received no diagnosis or no adjustment disorder diagnosis, suggesting clinical improvement since a decision for evacuation was made. |

**Health Effects of Military Service on Women Veterans**

| Author | Sample Characteristics | Sample Size | Design/Objective | Main Measures | Main Findings |
|---|---|---|---|---|---|
| Seal; 2009[32] | OIF and OEF Veterans who were first-time users of VA health care after their OIF and OEF military service from April 1, 2002 through March 31, 2008 | 289,328 | Observational; To investigate longitudinal trends and risk factors for mental health diagnoses among Iraq and Afghanistan Veterans | Prevalence of mental health diagnoses | • Of 289,328 Iraq and Afghanistan Veterans, 106,726 (36.9%) received mental health diagnoses; 62,929 (21.8%) were diagnosed with PTSD and 50,432 (17.4%) with depression.<br><br>• Adjusted 2-year prevalence rates of PTSD increased 4 to 7 times after the invasion of Iraq.<br><br>• Active duty Veterans younger than 25 years had higher rates of PTSD and alcohol and drug use disorder diagnoses compared with active duty Veterans older than 40 years (adjusted relative risk = 2.0 and 4.9, respectively).<br><br>• Women were at higher risk for depression than were men, but men had over twice the risk for drug use disorders.<br><br>• Greater combat exposure was associated with higher risk for PTSD. |
| Seal; 2010[35] | National subgroup of OEF and OIF Veterans who received VA health care services between April 1, 2002 and March 31, 2008 | 84,972 | Observational; To evaluate OEF and OIF Veterans' utilization of VA mental health services, looking at 3 main factors: predisposing, enabling, and need factors | VA mental health services utilization and the intensity of VA mental health services utilization | • Of 49,425 Veterans with newly diagnosed PTSD, only 9.5% attended 9 or more VA mental health sessions in 15 weeks or less in the first year of diagnosis.<br><br>• Engagement in 9 or more VA treatment sessions for PTSD within 15 weeks varied by predisposing variables (age and gender), enabling variables (clinic of first mental health diagnosis and distance from VA facility), and need (type and complexity of mental health diagnoses).<br><br>• Only a minority of Iraq and Afghanistan Veterans with new PTSD diagnoses received a recommended number and intensity of VA mental health treatment sessions within the first year of diagnosis. |
| Sherman; 2005[54] | Sample Veterans (and their female partners) who served in the Vietnam War, had a diagnosis of PTSD and service-connected disability for PTSD, participated in the PTSD program, and current cohabitation with a female partner recruited from two VA medical centers | Females 72 | Observational; To perform an initial needs assessment of Vietnam Veterans with combat-related post-traumatic stress disorder (PTSD) and to assess the partners' current rates of treatment use. | Partner treatment experiences and ratings of treatment needs; partners' assessment of her need for individual treatment and the partner's appraisal of family treatment being extremely important (yes/no). | Although large majorities of partners rated individual (64%) and family therapy (78%) to help cope with PTSD in the family as extremely or very important, only 28% had received any mental health care in the previous six months. Significant predictors of desire for individual treatment included partner's anxiety and patient-partner contact, and partner's age and severity of the patient's PTSD symptoms were significant predictors of family treatment. The most commonly requested service was a women-only group. |

**Health Effects of Military Service on Women Veterans**

| Author | Sample Characteristics | Sample Size | Design/Objective | Main Measures | Main Findings |
|---|---|---|---|---|---|
| Stecker; 2007[55] | VA national databases were used to identify Veterans receiving IOP substance use treatment, and Veterans with substance use disorders attending primary care but not in treatment. | Females 247 Males 8,082 | Observational; To investigate gender differences among Veterans receiving intensive outpatient (IOP) substance use treatment in a national VA sample and to compare women attending IOP with women with substance use disorders in VA primary care. | Psychiatric and medical conditions that co-occur with substance use disorder | Stigma was portrayed as a major disadvantage to treatment seeking. Yet most participants indicated that people would be supportive of treatment seeking. Reducing symptoms was a major advantage to care. Barriers included pride, not being able to ask for help, and not being able to admit to having a problem. |
| Street; 2009[34] | Literature review on gender-relevant issues among OEF/OIF female Veterans | N/A | Systematic review/meta-analysis; To highlight emerging issues relevant to the development of PTSD among women deployed to Iraq and Afghanistan | Combat experiences in Iraq and Afghanistan, sexual assault and sexual harassment, exposure to other interpersonal stressors, the role of premilitary and postmilitary interpersonal trauma, homecoming readjustment | Women are approximately twice as likely as their male counterparts to be diagnosed with PTSD. However, there are also indications that the gender-specific risk of PTSD differs substantially by type of traumatic event. |
| Wells; 2010[25] | Participants in the first panel of Millennium Cohort Study 2001-2006 who completed baseline and follow-up questionnaires and met inclusion criteria | 40,219 | Observational; To investigate relations between deployment and new-onset depression among US service members recently deployed | Comparison of new-onset depression by deployment status and gender | • Deployed men and women with combat exposures had the highest onset of depression, followed by those not deployed and those deployed without combat exposure.<br>• Combat –deployed men and women were at increased risk for new-onset depression compared with nondeployed men and women (men: adjusted oddos ration [AOR]=1.32; 95% CI=1.13, 1.54; women: AOR=2.13; 95% CI=1.70, 2.65).<br>• Conversely, deployment without combat exposures led to decreased risk for new-onset depression compared with those who did not deploy (men: AOR=0.66; 95% CI=0.53, 0.83; women: AOR=0.65; 95% CI=0.47, 0.89). |

**Health Effects of Military Service on Women Veterans**

| Author | Sample Characteristics | Sample Size | Design/Objective | Main Measures | Main Findings |
|---|---|---|---|---|---|
| Wojcik; 2010[30] | All U.S. Army soldiers deployed from September 2001 (OEF) and September 2002 (OEF) through December 2004 | 473,964 | Observational; To examine the magnitude and characteristics of mental disorder hospitalizations among U.S. Army soldiers deployed in Iraq and Afghanistan through December 2004 | Relative risks of mental disorder admissions in OIF and in OEF, attempted suicide/self-inflicted-related admissions | • There were a total of 1,948 psychiatric hospitalizations of deployed soldiers.<br>• The most common mental problems were mood, adjustment, anxiety disorders (including PTSD).<br>• Relative risk (RR) of mental disorders ranged from 1.6 to 3 for females and 2 to 6 for enlisted soldiers compared to their counterparts.<br>• Younger soldiers had 30-60% higher substance abuse disorders.<br>• Combat units in Iraq demonstrated higher risk of any mental disorder and anxiety problems compared to combat support units.<br>• Younger women had the highest incidence of attempted suicide/self-inflicted injuries. |
| Zivin; 2007[22] | National sample from the VA's National Registry for Depression (NARDEP) from April 1, 1999 to September 30, 2004 | 807,694 | Observational; To report clinical and demographic factors associated with suicide among depressed Veterans in an attempt to determine what characteristics identified Veterans at high risk for suicide | Suicide, and association with patient age, race, gender, substance abuse diagnosis, diagnosis of PTSD, Hispanic ethnicity, treatment location, prior VA hospitalization, service connection, and baseline medical comorbidity. | • Of 807,694 Veterans meeting study criteria, 1683 (0.21%) committed suicide during follow-up.<br>• Increased suicide risks were observed among male, younger, and non-Hispanic White patients.<br>• Veterans without service-connected disabilities, with inpatient psychiatric hospitalizations in the year prior to their qualifying depression diagnosis, with comorbid substance use, and living in the southern or western United States were also at higher risk.<br>• Posttraumatic stress disorder (PTSD) with comorbid depression was associated with lower suicide rates, and younger depressed Veterans with PTSD had a higher suicide rate than did older depressed Veterans with PTSD.<br>• Unlike the general population, older and younger Veterans are more prone to suicide than are middle-aged Veterans. |

43

| Author | Sample Characteristics | Sample Size | Design/Objective | Main Measures | Main Findings |
|---|---|---|---|---|---|
| Zouris; 2008[51] | Review of hospitalization data from OIF for casualties monitored by TRANSCOM Regulating and Command and Control Evacuation system (TRAC2ES) and Joint Patient Tracking Application (JPTA) that monitors all branches of the US Armed Forces in theatre of operations | Females 1,305 Males 11,766 | Observational; To describe the distribution of evacuated wounded in action (WIA) and Disease and Nonbattle Injury (DNBI) casualties sustained during the Major Combat Phase (OIF-1) and the Support and Stability Phase (OIF-2) of OIF involving the US Army and Marines | Primary ICD-9 diagnoses, gender, service were obtained, and casualties were classified as WIA or DNBI, subcategories of ICD-9 diagnoses were also created | The majority of casualties were DNBI (75%), Army personnel (83.5%) and were male (90%). Disease and nonbattle injury ICD-9 distributions differed by gender. The proportion of nonbattle injuries was significantly higher among men. Subcategories more common among women than men included neoplasms, mental disorders, diseases of the blood, respiratory, and genitourinary symptoms. |

www.ingramcontent.com/pod-product-compliance
Lightning Source LLC
Chambersburg PA
CBHW081624170526
45166CB00009B/3098